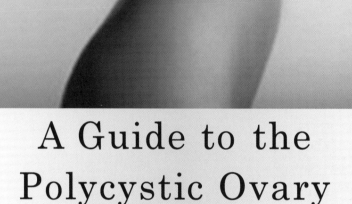

PROFESSOR GABOR KOVACS & JANE SMITH

A Guide to the Polycystic Ovary

Its Effects on Health and Fertility

t*f*m Publishing Ltd.

Acknowledgement

The authors wish to thank Professor Kovacs' secretary, Penny Heath, for all her help during the preparation of the book and for typing the manuscript.

tfm Publishing Limited
Castle Hill Barns
Harley
Nr Shrewsbury
SY5 6LX, UK.
Tel: +44 (0)1952 510061; Fax: +44 (0)1952 510192
E-mail: nikki@tfmpublishing.co.uk; Web site: www.tfmpublishing.co.uk

Design and layout: Nikki Bramhill
Original cover design: Deborah Snibson, Modern Art Production Group

First published in Australia 2001
by Hill of Content Publishing Pty Ltd
86 Bourke Street, Melbourne 3000
Tel: 03 9662 2282; Fax: 03 9662 2527
Email: hocpub@collinsbooks.com.au

Copyright © G. Kovacs 2002, J. Smith 2002
ISBN 1 903378 06 0

Printed by Ebenezer Baylis & Son Ltd., The Trinity Press, London Road, Worcester, WR5 2JH, UK. Tel: +44 (0)1905 357979; Fax: +44 (0)1905 354919.

Contents

Contents

Contents

One

Introduction

Historical background

In 1935, two doctors in the USA - Irving Stein and Michael Leventhal - published a report of surgery they had performed on a group of seven women with irregular or absent ovulation (anovulation) who had infrequent periods, increased hair growth on their face, arms, chest and abdomen, and were overweight. The operation - a major surgical procedure called wedge resection, which involves opening the abdomen to remove a slice of the ovary - resulted in all of the women ovulating successfully and two becoming pregnant. The syndrome identified in this group of women was originally called Stein-Leventhal syndrome, but is now more commonly known as polycystic ovary syndrome (PCOS), due to the presence on the surface of the ovaries of numerous small cysts, which have developed from follicles that have failed to mature.

Although documented references to polycystic ovary syndrome originate from the report of Stein and Leventhal in 1935, a literature search reveals that it may have been described very much earlier. In 1721, an Italian called Vallisneri wrote of: 'Young married peasant women, moderately obese and infertile, with two larger than normal ovaries, bumpy and shiny, whitish, just like pigeon eggs'; and in 1844, Chereau referred to hardening of the tissues of the ovary (known as sclerosis).

Polycystic ovaries and polycystic ovary syndrome

The first distinction that needs to be made is between polycystic ovaries and polycystic ovary syndrome. The former purely describes the appearance of the ovaries, as inspected from the outside during surgery (see page 4) or as visualized on an ultrasound examination (see page 19). If the symptoms caused by the presence of excessive male hormone are also present, the syndrome is diagnosed. The commonest of these symptoms is menstrual irregularity, or infrequent or even totally absent periods (amenorrhoea). Other common signs of excessive male hormone circulation (called androgenization) include the presence of pimples or acne, excessive hair growth, especially around the navel, nipples or face (called hirsutism), or hair loss of crown-pattern baldness (alopecia). Many women with polycystic ovary syndrome also have abnormal metabolism, causing them to be overweight, especially around the waist. This can be assessed by measuring their body mass index (BMI, see page 107) and waist:hip ratio.

Women with polycystic ovary syndrome may have varying combinations and degrees of all these abnormalities. The syndrome involves a wide spectrum of symptoms and therefore deciding whether or not a woman has polycystic ovary syndrome can be difficult. The patients first described by Stein and Leventhal in 1935 were all at the very severe end of this spectrum.

Even the diagnosis on ultrasound examination can be controversial. The ultrasound criteria for the diagnosis of polycystic ovaries are discussed in detail in Chapter 4. It is sufficient to state here that, even amongst experts, there is still no agreement on how large the ovary has to be or on how many cysts have to be present before the diagnosis of polycystic ovaries is made. To complicate matters further, there are women in whom one ovary has a typical polycystic appearance while the other is either normal or only borderline. It is therefore not surprising that different studies are difficult to compare.

How common are polycystic ovaries?

This is a difficult question to answer. It depends not only on which population of patients has been studied, but also on the diagnostic criteria used to define whether or not the ovaries are polycystic.

Despite these reservations, several studies have looked at populations of volunteers, women from the electoral roll and women attending general practices, and have carried out examinations of their ovaries by ultrasound and questioned them about symptoms. The first such study involved hospital employees in London and reported an incidence of polycystic ovaries of 23%, with some symptoms of excessive male hormone secretion being found in three out of four women. Even when women were selected from the electoral roll in Auckland, New Zealand, one in five were found to have the ultrasound appearance of polycystic ovaries, and over half of these had some signs of polycystic ovary syndrome. If groups of women with irregular periods are looked at, up to 90% will have polycystic ovaries at ultrasound. Similarly, when women with increased facial and body hair are screened, about 90% will have polycystic ovaries, as will three out of four women with acne. It has also been suggested by some studies that women with recurrent miscarriage or early pregnancy loss after in-vitro fertilization (see Chapter 12) have an increased incidence of polycystic ovaries. However, not all studies support this hypothesis, and additional research is needed to evaluate this further.

The pathological appearance of polycystic ovaries

Polycystic ovaries, when looked at with the naked eye at operation or after surgical removal, are typically enlarged and rounded (Figure 1.1, page 4). In one study, they were three times the size of the ovaries of a control group of women. The surface of the ovary is usually oyster-white, smooth and thickened, giving the appearance of a capsule or outer skin. On closer inspection, small cysts may be visible under the surface and, when the ovary is cut in half, the cut surface shows numerous, small, peripheral cysts, usually less than 10 mm in diameter, and the inner portion of the ovary has increased fibrous tissue (Figure 1.2, page 4).

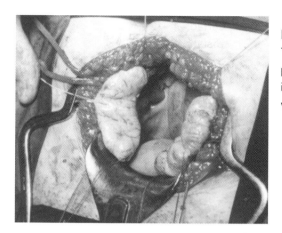

Figure 1.1
The appearance of the polycystic ovary, showing its enlarged, rounded, white outer surface.

Figure 1.2
The cut surface of the polycystic ovary, showing numerous, small, peripheral cysts set in the fibrous tissue.

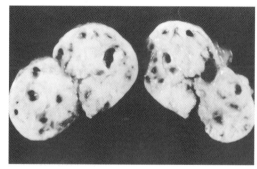

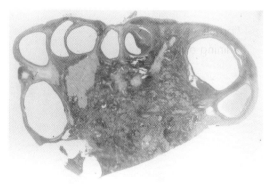

Figure 1.3
The microscopic appearance of the polycystic ovary, showing numerous follicular cysts around its periphery.

Illustrations reproduced by permission Cambridge University Press.

Microscopic examination of the surface of the ovary reveals increased development of fibrous tissue (fibrosis) on the outer rim. Although the follicles of women with polycystic ovaries appear to be no different from those of normal women, they are present in increased numbers (Figure 1.3). Microscopic examination also shows that there is a lack of the bodies found in the ovary after the rupture of the follicles (the corpora lutea), or of follicles at other stages of early development, and the numerous peripherally placed follicles appear trapped in fibrous tissue. When individual cysts are examined, they are found to have a thinner layer of cells than normal follicles.

It is interesting to note that the microscopic appearance of the ovaries of young girls prior to puberty and during the first few years of menstruation may be similar to that of polycystic ovaries.

In summary, the following are the features of polycystic ovary syndrome as seen on pathological examination:

- enlargement of the whole ovary,
- thickened capsule,
- increased number of small cysts under the capsule,
- absence of follicles that have ovulated or are in the process of maturing,
- thickening and increased fibrosis of the inner surface of the ovary,
- decreased thickness of the lining of each cyst.

T w o

The structure and function of the female genital organs

Before going into the details of polycystic ovary syndrome, it is useful to have some understanding of the structure of the female genital organs and their function.

The internal genital organs

The internal genital organs consist of a womb (uterus), two fallopian tubes, two ovaries and a vagina, the external opening of which is surrounded by the vulva (Figure 2.1).

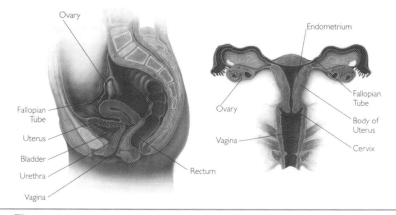

Figure 2.1 The female genital organs. (Reproduced by permission.)

THE OVARIES

The two ovaries are oval organs, which, after puberty, are usually about the size of a walnut (approximately 3 cm long). Each ovary is situated near the open end of a fallopian tube (see below). The function of the ovaries is to produce hormones and eggs, known as ova (singular, ovum).

Within a newborn baby girl there is a complete complement of several thousand ova, each smaller than a grain of salt. Each ovum is surrounded by a blister-like follicle. Although the ova themselves do not increase in size after puberty, follicles mature and enlarge each month, and their ova become surrounded by fluid. Usually, a whole crop of follicles starts to develop, but only one becomes the leading follicle, the one that is ultimately released at ovulation. This leading follicle somehow suppresses its neighbours so that, in a normal cycle, only one oocyte is released, thereby avoiding multiple pregnancies most of the time. This process has not developed in most other animals, which is why they have litters, whereas humans usually only have single babies. Ovulation normally occurs monthly, in the middle of the menstrual cycle throughout a woman's reproductive life.

The follicle usually takes 10-16 days to mature and, at ovulation, ruptures and releases its ovum. (If we imagine the follicle as being similar to a hen's egg, the ovum is equivalent to the yolk.) The ovum then passes into the adjacent fallopian tube and the remains of the follicle (which, in the hen's egg, would have been the shell and some of the egg white) form a yellow structure known as the corpus luteum ('yellow body' in Latin). Whereas the developing follicle produces only oestrogen, the corpus luteum produces some oestrogen but also progesterone. The hormone progesterone is essential for preparing the lining of the womb for pregnancy.

THE FALLOPIAN TUBES

The two fallopian tubes (each of which is about 10 cm long) have complicated and intricate functions.

7

- They are responsible for picking up the ovum from the ovarian surface after ovulation, a process that is performed at the open end of each tube by finger-like structures called fimbriae.
- Tiny hair-like structures (called cilia) on their inner surface help waft the ovum towards the uterus.
- The lumen of the tube also provides a passageway for the last few hundred or so sperm as they head towards the ovum, with the aim of fertilizing it.
- They provide an environment in which the ovum meets and is joined by the sperm - in the process known as fertilization. This normally occurs within the outer third of the fallopian tube and the fertilized ovum then passes down the remainder of the tube towards the uterus.
- The passage of the fertilized ovum (now called the embryo) is dependent on the healthy functioning of the fallopian tube.
- They provide nutrition for the rapidly developing early embryo.

THE UTERUS

The uterus (or womb) is a muscular organ, about the size and shape of a pear. It consists of two parts: the body (corpus) and the neck (cervix). The fallopian tubes open into its upper corners, the part above which is known as the fundus.

The uterus has a muscular outer layer (the myometrium) and an inner, soft, honeycomb-like layer (the endometrium). It is rich in blood vessels and its main function is to provide a protected environment in which the embryo (which then becomes the fetus) can develop. The muscle tissue changes little month to month, but the endometrium goes through a cycle of thickening, increased vascularity and, in the absence of a pregnancy, shedding. It is the shedding of the endometrium that is responsible for the menstrual loss during a woman's menstrual period, together with bleeding from the many blood vessels of the endometrium. If fertilization occurs and an embryo enters the uterine cavity, the endometrium provides a suitable surface for its implantation.

THE VAGINA

The vagina is a muscular canal extending from the uterus to the vulva. It is usually about 8 cm long and very elastic. It forms a connection between the neck of the womb (the cervix) and the outside of the body. During intercourse, it helps the penis to deposit sperm near the cervical opening.

Menstruation

The first menstruation for a young woman is known as the menarche. It normally occurs in girls between the ages of about 10 and 16, although this age varies in different parts of the world, being partly dependent on the girl attaining a minimum body weight, and therefore on her level of nutrition. Although the menstrual cycle may be irregular to begin with, it usually settles into a pattern after a couple of years.

At puberty, the hypothalamus in the brain starts to produce the hormones that stimulate the pituitary gland to release other hormones into the body's circulation. These pituitary hormones include follicle-stimulating hormone (FSH), whose role it is to stimulate follicles, and luteinizing hormone (LH), whose role it is to trigger ovulation and thus produce a corpus luteum, both of which act directly on the ovaries.

As the level of FSH increases, follicles in the ovaries start to mature and to produce the hormone oestrogen. This then triggers the release of LH, which, in turn, triggers ovulation (Figure 2.2, page 10). After the follicle matures and releases its ovum, it collapses, forming a corpus luteum.

Unless the released ovum is fertilized and implants in the endometrium within hours of ovulation, the corpus luteum dies within about 10-14 days and the levels of progesterone and oestrogen fall and, consequently, the endometrium cannot be maintained. Approximately 14 days after ovulation, the endometrium therefore breaks down, its blood vessels rupture and menstrual bleeding occurs. A new menstrual cycle begins as

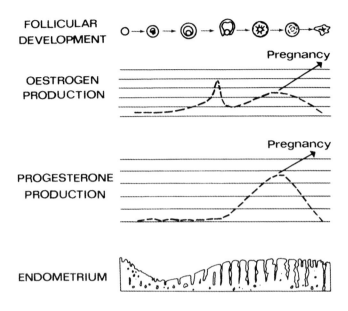

Figure 2.2 The menstrual cycle, showing hormonal changes and follicular and endometrial development.

FSH is once again secreted. Menstruation can therefore be viewed as a failure of the ovulatory cycle with no resultant pregnancy.

However, if the ovum is fertilized, the early embryo produces the hormone human chorionic gonadotrophin (HCG), which 'rescues' the corpus luteum and enables it to continue to secrete oestrogen and progesterone. These hormones prevent the lining of the uterus being shed so that the embryo can implant and develop a placenta. The corpus luteum persists for up to 8-10 weeks, after which the hormones are secreted by the placenta. The measurement of HCG in the blood or urine is used as a pregnancy test to show that conception has occurred.

Three

Symptoms and signs

The term *polycystic ovary* refers to the appearance of the ovary on ultrasound. A diagnosis of *polycystic ovary syndrome* requires the presence of clinical symptoms of male hormone excess (androgenization) - menstrual irregularity and/or increased hair growth, acne and obesity.

Introduction

Population studies have shown that the ovaries of up to 25% of women are polycystic. Many of these women have no symptoms, but often there is an increase in the secretion of male hormones, resulting in acne and increased hair growth. Although this may be associated with menstrual irregularity, this is not the predominant symptom for many women, who therefore may be seen by a skin specialist rather than by a gynaecologist.

The different aspects of polycystic ovary syndrome can be represented as three circles, showing the ultrasonic, clinical and biochemical changes that occur (Figure 3.1, page 12). Although some women will demonstrate all three aspects of the syndrome, others may only experience one or two of them.

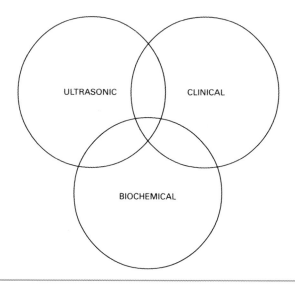

Figure 3.1 Polycystic ovary syndrome.

In fully manifest cases, women have infrequent ovulation and periods, and symptoms associated with an increase in male hormone secretion are obvious. The polycystic nature of the ovaries is apparent on ultrasound (see page 19). The changes related to the increase in male hormone secretion are caused by biochemical abnormalities, which can be detected by blood tests. These abnormalities include an excess ratio of luteinizing hormone (LH) to follicle-stimulating hormone (FSH) and increased levels of the male hormones androstenedione and testosterone.

With the discovery of these abnormalities has come the understanding that polycystic ovary syndrome is not just a disease of the reproductive system (manifestations of which are easily remedied by treatment with fertility tablets, injections or surgery), but is a more widespread disease, affecting the metabolism of the whole body. Consequently, it is important to look at this condition in a more holistic way.

Weight and fat distribution

The classical woman with polycystic ovary syndrome is described as being overweight. This tendency towards obesity is apparent in 30-50% of women with the condition. Obesity is defined by calculating the woman's body mass index (BMI, see page 61). Furthermore, the fat is distributed in such a way that there is an increased waist measurement, giving rise to what is called central obesity or an apple shape (in contrast to the more usual pear shape). Central obesity can be quantified in terms of the waist:hip ratio.

Insulin resistance

Recently, as more detailed investigations of women with polycystic ovary syndrome have been carried out, it has become recognized that this condition is often associated with an abnormality of carbohydrate metabolism known as insulin resistance. Insulin resistance leads to an increased requirement for the secretion of insulin by the pancreas in order to metabolize the body's blood sugars and keep them within the normal range. When the pancreas can no longer secrete sufficient amounts of insulin to maintain the body's sugar levels in the normal range, persistently raised blood sugar levels - diabetes - develop.

The measurement of insulin resistance is difficult, and involves both insulin and glucose levels, and methods are currently restricted to research studies and are not yet readily available.

Diabetes

Type I diabetes usually develops in childhood and needs to be treated with insulin. Type II diabetes (known as non-insulin-dependent diabetes mellitus - NIDDM) develops in adults and can usually be adequately managed with diet and oral medication to counteract the insulin resistance. Women with polycystic ovary syndrome tend to develop NIDDM, the criteria for the diagnosis of which are summarized in Table

3.1. However, many women with polycystic ovary syndrome have some degree of insulin resistance in the absence of frank diabetes.

GLUCOSE TOLERANCE TEST

Frank diabetes can be diagnosed by a special blood test called a glucose tolerance test (GTT). Prior to attending the clinic for this test, the woman must fast for at least 8 hours. A sample of blood is taken to measure her basal (fasting) blood sugar level and she is then given a glass of sweet cordial to drink, which contains a measured amount of glucose (50 mg). Her resultant blood sugar levels are then measured after 1 and 2 hours. If the pancreas is functioning normally and is able to produce sufficient insulin, the blood sugar will not reach excessively high levels and will return to normal within 2 hours. If the sugar levels remain significantly elevated, insulin resistance and diabetes are present.

Table 3.1 Oral glucose tolerance test (GTT) values for diagnosing various categories of hyperglycaemia.

	Venous plasma glucose (mmol/L)
Diabetes	
Fasting	>7.0
2-hour GTT	>11.0
Impaired glucose tolerance	
Fasting	<7.0
2-hour GTT	>7.7 and <11.0
Impaired fasting glucose	
Fasting	>6.1 and <7.0
2-hour GTT	<7.8

Atherosclerosis

Apart from the evidence that women with polycystic ovary syndrome have insulin resistance and consequently an increased risk of developing diabetes, there is also some suggestion of an increased risk of thickening of the arteries (atherosclerosis) and consequent heart attacks. It is well recognized that the most serious complication of diabetes is its deleterious effect on the blood vessels.

RAISED CHOLESTEROL AND TRIGLYCERIDES

Sometimes, affected women also have raised levels of the body fats cholesterol and triglycerides. It has been recognized for the last 20 years or so that raised levels of both cholesterol and triglycerides predispose to thickening of and damage to the lining of arteries. This results in decreased blood flow to the organs that the artery supplies, and causes a lack of blood supply and oxygen. If the level of blood flow becomes critically impaired, the end organ is damaged. If the affected arteries supply the heart (the coronary arteries), this causes coronary occlusion, known as a 'heart attack'. If the arteries to the brain are blocked, this causes strokes. Blockage of the arteries to the legs causes muscle pain on walking. It is for these reasons that people are encouraged to decrease their cholesterol intake by eating low-fat diets and to use medications if their cholesterol level is high.

Increased male hormone effects

The hormonal abnormalities seen in women with polycystic ovaries result in a series of complex biochemical processes. The raised levels of LH give rise to an increased secretion of the male-type hormone androstenedione and a subsequent increase in circulating testosterone.

This is further exacerbated because of the effect of the raised level of insulin, which causes the liver to decrease its secretion of sex hormone-binding globulin (SHBG), which normally binds to, and inactivates, testosterone. The lower levels of SHBG, and therefore the smaller amount available for binding to testosterone, lead to an increase in the circulating level of active, unbound testosterone. The effect is therefore an increase in the amount of chemically active male hormones - increased secretion and decreased binding.

15

Increased hair growth

One of the most obvious effects of increased male hormone activity in the body is the increase in body hair that results from stimulation of the hair follicles. Until the 1960s, when chemicals became available to counteract male hormones, the treatment for increased hair growth was purely cosmetic. The first chemical treatment was a tablet called spironolactone (normally used to treat persistent swelling of the tissues known as oedema). It was followed by a specific anti-androgen tablet called cyproterone acetate and, more recently, by flutamide. All of these have been used successfully to treat acne and increased hair growth.

Pimples and acne

One of the commonest manifestations of polycystic ovary syndrome is pimples or acne resulting from the effects of the increased circulating levels and increased activity of the male hormones on the skin and sweat glands. This is described in detail in Chapter 9.

Infertility and anovulation

Although women may simply put up with the unpleasant side-effects of polycystic ovary syndrome, they often need to seek medical advice when inadequate ovulation leads to an inability to conceive. Fortunately, this aspect of polycystic ovary syndrome can now usually be successfully treated. In addition to the surgical technique of wedge resection mentioned in Chapter 1, fertility tablets (clomiphene citrate) and injections of FSH (gonadotrophins) became available during the 1960s. These treatments usually result in ovulation and rapid conception, and are discussed in detail in Chapter 10.

Four

Diagnostic techniques

With further developments in reproductive medicine and the availability of an oral tablet (clomiphene citrate) in 1961, it became possible to treat women with irregular periods and infrequent ovulation using medication rather than surgery. However, the investigations carried out were usually minimal and it was not determined whether the women being treated had polycystic ovaries. Further refinement of the diagnosis of polycystic ovaries came with the widespread availability of ultrasound examination (see below) and, particularly, with the ability to perform scans through the vagina.

Radiology

Even before ultrasound became available, a radiological technique was developed in the 1930s that allowed a diagnosis to be made without the need to open the abdomen and actually look at and feel the ovaries. This technique involves injecting air into the abdominal cavity to outline the ovaries and uterus and then identifying the polycystic ovaries on x-ray, the diagnosis being made on the basis of the size of the ovarian shadow as compared to the uterine shape.

Biochemical techniques

With improvements in biochemical techniques, including the development of radio-immunoassay during the 1970s, the emphasis changed to a biochemical diagnosis of polycystic ovaries. Increased concentrations of luteinizing hormone (LH) and testosterone were thought to be essential prerequisites for this diagnosis. The ratio of LH to follicle-stimulating hormone (FSH) - which is secreted by the brain but measured in the blood - was also considered to be an important diagnostic criterion. The ratio thought necessary for a diagnosis of polycystic ovaries to be made has changed over the years, but is currently 2.5:1. Increased blood levels of the male hormones testosterone and androstenedione are also often associated with polycystic ovary syndrome (see above) and have been measured to make the diagnosis.

However, the weakness of measuring the LH level as a diagnostic tool lies in the fact that this hormone is secreted in a pulsatile fashion into the bloodstream, resulting in constantly varying levels, and therefore potentially misleading results when a spot test is done.

Ultrasonography

The real breakthrough in the diagnosis of polycystic ovaries came with the development of ultrasound techniques (or ultrasonography). Ultrasound is a non-invasive, painless, simple, relatively cheap and repeatable measurement of ovarian size, which also shows the number of follicles present.

An ultrasound scan involves passing high-frequency sound waves (similar to radar) into the body. When the sound waves meet a solid object within the body cavity, they are reflected back like an echo and a computer processes the waves and builds up a picture, which is displayed on a screen.

There has been considerable debate about the ultrasound diagnostic criteria of what constitutes a polycystic ovary. However, the consensus seems to be that there should be 10-12 small follicles, 2-6 mm in diameter, distributed around the periphery of the ovary, together with an increase in ovarian volume greater than 5.5 cm^3 (Figure 4.1). Although both transabdominal and transvaginal methods have been used to assess the ovary, there is no doubt that detection rates are much higher when transvaginal ultrasound is used.

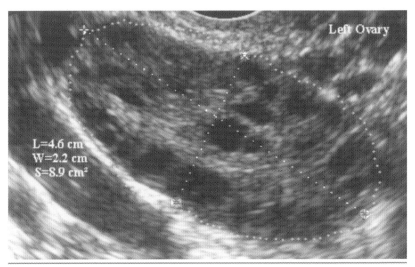

Figure 4.1 A polycystic ovary as seen on ultrasound. (Reproduced by permission Cambridge University Press.)

For an abdominal scan, a special jelly-like substance is smeared onto the abdomen, and a probe is gently moved over it. The vaginal scan is done by gently inserting a small probe (about the size of one or two fingers) into the vagina.

Before the development of ultrasonography, polycystic ovaries were diagnosed at operation either by laparotomy (opening the abdomen) or by laparoscopy (introducing a surgical instrument containing a telescope through a small incision in the body wall). However, since the 1980s, ultrasonography has become the recognized method of diagnosis.

Using ultrasonography, through either the vagina or the abdomen, the size and shape of the ovaries can be measured and the internal structure can be visualized.

19

THE ULTRASOUND EXAMINATION

This usually consists of both a transabdominal and a transvaginal examination. The abdominal examination allows a panoramic view of the contents of the pelvis to be obtained, as well as a good overall view of the uterus and the ovaries. In order to visualize the ovaries properly with a transabdominal scan, the patient has to have a full bladder, which can be achieved either by drinking lots of fluids or by the insertion of a catheter and expansion of the bladder with water. However, abdominal ultrasound gives a fairly limited view of the inside of the ovaries, which can be better assessed by transvaginal scanning.

Transvaginal scanning is usually performed after abdominal scanning unless the patient is a virgin or does not wish to have a vaginal examination.

There can be other situations in which there are multiple follicles within the ovary, such as during puberty, when there is anovulation due to other causes, or in the early phase of an ovulatory cycle. It is therefore important to differentiate true polycystic ovaries - which are larger and often more spherical in shape - from these multi-follicular ovaries.

Ultrasound examination allows:

◆ calculation of the ovarian area and/or volume,
◆ confirmation of increased roundness (when the ovarian width to ovarian length ratio is increased),
◆ measurement of the width of the uterine fundus and the length of the ovary to establish whether there is a decreased uterine width to ovarian length ratio.

The internal morphology of the ovary is also inspected, the key features that are looked for being a number of small, echo-less regions (cysts) less than 10 mm in diameter within the ovary. These cysts are usually at the periphery of the ovary rather than being uniformly distributed. The inner (stromal) area of the ovary appears white on ultrasound scanning and has increased density due to its increased thickness.

20

THREE-DIMENSIONAL ULTRASOUND

A further refinement of scanning is three-dimensional ultrasound, which uses a computer program to scan the ovarian shape in three dimensions. The data collected enable an accurate calculation to be made of the ovarian volume. However, this technique does not offer any other advantages.

DOPPLER ULTRASOUND

Doppler ultrasound is a refinement of ultrasonography that has recently become available. It has the advantage of enabling blood flow to be detected as changes in colour. When used as part of an ultrasound examination, colour Doppler enables the degree of vascularization within the ovarian stroma to be assessed. The blood flow through the major vessels can also be measured by what is called the pulsatility index.

However, the study of ovarian vascularization using the Doppler technique is highly subjective and neither of these techniques has greatly added to the imaging diagnosis of polycystic ovaries. Although the increased stromal component of polycystic ovaries generally seems to be accompanied by increased vascularization, the measurements for patients with polycystic ovaries usually overlap those for normal patients.

SUMMARY

Ultrasonography is the tool of choice to diagnose polycystic ovaries. However, much of the information obtained on ultrasound scanning is qualitative, depending to some extent on the 'eye of the beholder' rather than being unequivocally quantitative. It is also difficult to define clearly a control group of normal patients against whom the abnormalities of polycystic ovaries can be defined. Nevertheless, ultrasonography has widened the clinical spectrum of polycystic ovaries, with many women being diagnosed in the absence of any other clinical symptoms.

In a recent survey in Melbourne in which the wives of sterile men were assessed, over 23% of these apparently 'normal' women had ovaries classified as 'polycystic' on the above criteria.

Magnetic resonance imaging

Reports in the literature of the appearance of polycystic ovaries on magnetic resonance imaging (MRI) are still scarce.

MRI involves the use of a scanner in the form of a large, high-powered magnet. Following the injection of a contrast medium, the patient lies on a table, which passes through a tunnel containing the magnet. A computer then produces a picture of the ovaries.

This technique allows scans to be taken through the body in a number of planes and thus the shape of the ovary to be reconstructed. The external signs of polycystic ovaries are then easily analysed, with transverse sections showing the multitude of cysts within the ovarian periphery (microcysts). However, analysis of the thickened stroma of the ovaries is more difficult on MRI than on ultrasonography.

SUMMARY
MRI does not provide any extra information beyond that obtained by ultrasonography and is far more expensive. However, if ultrasonography is not possible or is unhelpful, particularly if transvaginal scanning cannot be carried out, MRI may have a place in the diagnosis of polycystic ovaries. Its most useful application is in scanning the ovaries to exclude the presence of a tumour that might be producing male hormone and masquerading as polycystic ovaries. This alternative diagnosis should be suspected if the ovarian shape is not symmetrical or if there is a circumscribed, localized abnormality.

Some people are unable to tolerate the whole scan because the tunnel makes them claustrophobic. As the procedure involves the use of a magnet, nothing made of metal should be taken into the scanning tunnel.

Five

The inheritance of polycystic ovary syndrome

It is now believed that a genetic factor is strongly implicated in this condition, as a high percentage of the female relatives of women with polycystic ovary syndrome also suffer from it and their male relatives show premature balding.

Genes and chromosomes

The genetic bases of many diseases are now well understood. It is estimated that humans have between 50,000 and 80,000 genes, as determined on the human genome, and that every individual carries a few 'bad genes'. All the genes are carried on chromosomes, which are double-stranded structures made up of DNA and contained within the nucleus of every cell in the body.

The chromosomes of every cell in a particular individual carry the same genetic information. Humans have 23 pairs of chromosomes, 22 of which are known as autosomes. The 23rd pair comprises the 'sex chromosomes'; these include one X and one Y chromosome in males and two X chromosomes in females. There are two genes for each characteristic of an individual, such as eye colour etc., one of which is inherited from the individual's mother and the other from the father. These two genes occur in identical places on the two chromosomes in a pair. If a condition is 'dominant', it will be manifest even if only one of the chromosomes carries the abnormal gene for it. However, for a 'recessive' condition to become manifest, the abnormal gene must be present on both chromosomes.

Chromosome numbers and shapes

It is possible to analyse the chromosomal complement (i.e. number and shape of the chromosomes) of individuals, which is known as their karyotype. An abnormality in the number of chromosomes present in an individual is called aneuploidy. An example of an aneuploidy is Down's syndrome, in which there is a total of 47 (rather than the normal 46) chromosomes in every cell. In a few conditions, parts of the genetic material of a chromosome are missing, which is called a deletion. For example, Y chromosome deletion appears to be associated with some types of male infertility involving a low sperm count.

Chromosome analysis studies have been carried out on women with polycystic ovaries. Although some of these have reported abnormalities of the X chromosome and of other chromosomes in a limited number of subjects, gross alterations of chromosome structure do not seem to be a feature of the inheritance of polycystic ovaries.

The study of hereditary diseases

Unlike other abnormalities for which the responsible genes have been identified (such as the hereditary bleeding disease haemophilia or the inherited anaemia-related disorder thalassaemia), polycystic ovary syndrome is not thought to be passed on by a single gene. Instead, it is likely to be linked to a combination of genes interacting with various environmental factors, the most important of which is probably the woman's body weight.

There are numerous problems associated with the study of the genetics of the inheritance of polycystic ovary syndrome, which account for the fact that its mode of inheritance is not yet completely understood. For example, because the condition mainly becomes apparent during the reproductive years, it is difficult to study several generations. There is also some debate about how it is manifested in male relatives, although the premature baldness mentioned above is one possibility that is favoured.

The other major problem in genetic studies involves the varying definitions of what constitutes a polycystic ovary and polycystic ovary syndrome, and the consequent difficulty of carrying out family studies. Nevertheless, some family studies have been attempted and reports of at least nine have been published in the medical literature. Not surprisingly, the conclusions drawn from these studies are varied, although the majority do seem to suggest that the condition has an autosomal dominant inheritance and can be inherited from either the maternal or paternal side. (An autosomal condition is one that is related to a gene carried on the autosomal chromosomes, rather than on the sex chromosomes.)

Another interesting approach to the study of the inheritance of polycystic ovary syndrome has involved twins. The involvement of identical twins is useful in studies of inheritance because they have identical genes and therefore any abnormal gene would be present in both of them. Although the number of twins studied is small, it is not unusual to find that one twin has polycystic ovary syndrome and the other does not. This finding further confuses the involvement of inheritance and emphasizes the influence of environmental factors.

Several small studies have shown clusters of women with polycystic ovaries within families. The first of these found that women with polycystic ovaries that had definitely been confirmed by wedge resection or by inspection with a telescope had a higher incidence of first-degree relatives with irregular periods than women in the general population. Another study selected women diagnosed as having polycystic ovary syndrome on the basis of increased hair growth. The women's responses to a postal questionnaire showed that their female first-degree relatives had a higher incidence of hirsutism and irregular periods and that their male relatives had a higher incidence of premature balding than would be expected by chance.

The results of a study involving the diagnosis of polycystic ovaries by ultrasound examination in symptomatic women, followed by the ultrasound examination of their first-degree relatives, showed that polycystic ovaries were diagnosed even more often than would have been expected for an autosomal dominant inherited disease.

Another study went further than just looking at ovarian appearance and at the symptoms of excess androgen secretion, by carrying out biochemical tests for insulin and blood concentrations of triglycerides (see page 15). It found that there was a higher than expected biochemical disturbance amongst the relatives of the women involved.

Another group studied the 155 sisters of 80 women with polycystic ovary syndrome, measuring their androgen levels and recording their menstrual patterns. About 25% of the sisters were found to have irregular menstrual cycles and raised androgen levels, and another 25% had raised androgen levels but regular cycles. This is further evidence for an autosomal dominant mode of inheritance for increased androgen production.

However, none of the family studies reported so far has convincingly established the mode of inheritance of polycystic ovaries or polycystic ovary syndrome, possibly because not enough families have been studied, or because of the uncertainty in determining which women were affected and the difficulties involved in tracking and categorizing their relatives.

Techniques used to determine inheritance

Molecular biology techniques are used for the analysis of genomic DNA from large numbers of families with one or more members who have been identified as having polycystic ovaries. The data are then compared to those from families without polycystic ovaries in an attempt to detect any over-representation of a specific candidate gene amongst the affected families. Several genes that may be responsible for causing polycystic ovary syndrome have been studied. However, these studies are subject to error and do not confirm that a specific gene causes the disease. Their findings may also be biased by the way in which the control population is selected. For example, the inclusion of women with unrecognized polycystic ovaries in the control population may result in misleading findings. It is therefore no surprise that conflicting results have been reported from different studies.

Factors that may indicate genetic inheritance

In order to understand the inheritance of the abnormality, some studies have focused on the various parameters that make up polycystic ovary syndrome. As the main symptoms are related to excessive male hormone secretion, abnormal carbohydrate metabolism and abnormalities of the secretion and regulation of gonadotrophin, the genes responsible for these factors have been studied.

EXCESSIVE MALE HORMONE SECRETION
As mentioned in Chapter 1, increased secretion of male-type hormones (androgens) is a frequent finding in women with polycystic ovary syndrome. The two main androgens involved are androstenedione and dihydroepiandrosterone (DHEA), both of which are metabolized to testosterone. The other active hormone in the circulation is dihydrotestosterone. About 50% of circulating testosterone usually comes from the ovaries or the adrenal glands, and 50% results from the conversion of androstenedione, especially in fatty tissue. Most women with polycystic ovary syndrome have raised levels of both testosterone and androstenedione, although there is a huge variation among them.

The complexity of this condition is highlighted by the surprising findings that women with infrequent periods but no signs of increased male hormone effects may have elevated levels of the relevant androgens in their blood, whereas other women with increased hair growth and acne may have normal levels of androgens. The symptoms experienced are probably a reflection of the varying sensitivity of the hair follicles to androgens in different individuals and also of the variable rates of clearance of these hormones from the circulation.

Another confounding factor is sex hormone-binding globulin (SHBG), which circulates in the bloodstream and binds both testosterone and dihydrotestosterone. As long as these hormones are bound, they do not have the ability to stimulate hair follicles. Therefore, anything that increases the level of SHBG in the circulation will result in an increase in the amount of these two hormones that is bound and thus a decrease in their active levels and peripheral effects.

A laboratory study by a group at St Mary's Hospital in London compared the production (in test tubes) of male hormones by cells from the ovarian follicles of women with polycystic ovary syndrome with that of cells from the ovaries of normal controls. It was found that hormone production was significantly increased in the cells from the women with polycystic ovary syndrome, suggesting that increased male hormone-producing activity is intrinsic to these cells.

ABNORMALITIES IN INSULIN SECRETION AND ACTION

It has been found that women with polycystic ovary syndrome have increased levels of insulin in their blood and insulin resistance compared to weight-matched controls (see Chapter 3). When the level of insulin secreted by the pancreas is no longer enough to maintain a normal level of sugar in the blood, diabetes and complications associated with raised levels of blood sugar develop. Consequently, the prevalence of impaired glucose tolerance in obese women with polycystic ovary syndrome is significantly greater than that of weight-matched controls (30% versus 10%), particularly in women in their thirties and forties. Furthermore, a follow-up study of post-menopausal women with polycystic ovary syndrome found a 15% prevalence of non-insulin-dependent diabetes mellitus (NIDDM), compared to 5% in a control group, suggesting that polycystic ovary syndrome is a major risk factor in the development of diabetes.

Potential candidate genes

The possible candidate genes that have been investigated include those involved with the synthesis of steroid hormones, including *CYP11A* (cholesterol side-chain cleavage gene), which alters androgen production, *CYP19* (the gene encoding P450 aromatase) and *CYP17* (17-hydroxylase-17,20-lysase gene). However, none of these has been confirmed as a likely candidate.

As insulin resistance and abnormality of insulin secretion seem to be part of polycystic ovary syndrome, genes related to insulin secretion and insulin function have also been studied. There is some evidence that part of the *insulin gene* called the VNTR (variable number tandem repeat) may contribute to the mechanism of insulin resistance, but this has not been confirmed. The insulin receptor gene has also been considered as a candidate, but is now discounted.

Because abnormally raised levels of luteinizing hormone are very common in women with polycystic ovaries, another potential candidate gene is one involved in gonadotrophin action and regulation. Consequently, the *follistatin gene* was considered, but its role has not yet been confirmed.

Conclusions

Polycystic ovary syndrome is a disorder of unknown cause, with clusters in families and probably a genetic component. The exact mode of inheritance is not yet understood, although clinical genetic studies have pointed to it being autosomal dominant, perhaps modified by environmental factors. Several potential candidate genes have been proposed, including *CYP11A*, the insulin gene and the follistatin gene, but none has been proven to be involved.

For a complete understanding of the inheritance of polycystic ovary syndrome, two types of studies will have to be successfully carried out.

1. The prevalence of the syndrome in the relatives (usually sisters) of affected women needs to be determined in an unbiased way in studies of appropriately selected populations.
2. Studies to test the linkage between polycystic ovary syndrome and candidate genes need to be undertaken in families with multiple subjects. Several genes have to be tested for, and care needs to be taken to ensure that a particular gene is not identified by chance.

As there is still debate about the effects of polycystic ovary syndrome in males, these studies should initially only involve women until significant evidence of linkage is found. The data can then be extended to male relatives with premature baldness.

S i x

Long-term effects

Up to one in four women may have polycystic ovaries and polycystic ovary syndrome (i.e. with metabolic disturbances in addition to the ultrasound findings). The syndrome is passed on in families, although, as explained in Chapter 5, its exact mode of inheritance is not clear. In recent years it has become apparent that polycystic ovary syndrome involves more than just irregular ovulation and infrequent periods. Because of the possible association of the genes responsible for polycystic ovary syndrome with the cholesterol-cleaving gene and the insulin gene, and because of the abnormalities of lipid and glucose metabolism in women with polycystic ovaries, there has been concern about possible implications other than the lack of ovulation.

Heavy periods

Although there is not a great deal of information about the long-term effects of polycystic ovary syndrome, there has been one long-term study from Sweden involving 33 women who were treated by wedge resection between 1956 and 1965. These women were compared to 130 control women who were matched for age at the time of study in 1987. The women were followed up for over two decades and it was found that the risk of requiring a hysterectomy to treat heavy periods was three times greater in the treated (polycystic ovary syndrome) women (21%) than in the control women (7%). A similar increased risk was also indicated in a study in New Zealand. It is therefore apparent that women with polycystic ovary syndrome are more likely to require hysterectomy than women who do not suffer from this condition.

Osteoporosis

There is no evidence of any increased osteoporosis (thinning of the bones) in women with polycystic ovary syndrome. Although women with this condition have irregular periods and hormonal abnormality due to their increased secretion of male-type hormones (androgens), their bone mineral density is maintained and osteoporosis does not develop.

Obesity

Women tend to put on a few kilograms of extra weight during the years leading up to their menopause. Women with polycystic ovary syndrome in the Swedish study mentioned above showed an overall weight decrease at this time, but maintained their central obesity (i.e. maintaining the deposition of fat around the waist) and a constant waist:hip ratio of about 0.8, giving them an 'apple shape' rather than the more usual female 'pear shape'. The control women in this study showed a decrease in their waist:hip ratio despite their weight gain, suggesting an increased deposition of fat on their hips.

It has long been recognized that excessive male hormone production leads to increased fat deposition around the waist, and that central obesity is associated with insulin resistance, an unfavourable lipid profile and an increased risk of cardiovascular disease. This is further circumstantial evidence that polycystic ovary syndrome constitutes a 'health hazard', especially for cardiovascular disease.

Insulin resistance and diabetes

Increased androgenic hormone levels are associated with insulin resistance, and insulin resistance is the underlying metabolic disorder in polycystic ovary syndrome, affected women having an increased risk of developing non-insulin-dependent diabetes mellitus (NIDDM).

Whereas obesity can also result in insulin resistance, women with polycystic ovary syndrome have repeatedly been shown to be insulin resistant to a greater degree than weight-matched controls. Non-obese women with polycystic ovary syndrome have also been shown to be insulin resistant.

Insulin resistance has been clearly demonstrated to be more common amongst women with polycystic ovary syndrome in two studies. The first is the Swedish study mentioned above, in which the incidence of NIDDM was almost five times higher in the women with polycystic ovary syndrome than it was in the controls (15% versus 3.2%). A weakness of this study was that it did not compare other risk factors such as body weight or shape between the two groups.

The second study is a large British study that analysed the death certificates of 786 women diagnosed as having polycystic ovary syndrome between 1930 and 1979. Diabetes was mentioned nearly four times as often as would have been expected. However, again in this study it was not possible to adjust for other risk factors for diabetes such as obesity, although obesity did seem to have an additive effect on insulin resistance.

When insulin resistance is present with normal pancreatic function, the pancreas simply has to work harder to make more insulin and keep the blood sugar levels normal. If the pancreas is unable to produce sufficient insulin, the blood sugar levels increase and diabetes develops. Therefore, there seems to be good evidence that women with polycystic ovaries or polycystic ovary syndrome do have an increased risk of diabetes (NIDDM) in their later years. In addition to the health risks related to the development of diabetes itself, there is also the concern that it is a clearly recognized risk factor for cardiovascular disease.

Lipid profiles

Another risk factor for cardiovascular disease is the presence of raised levels of certain fats (lipids) in the blood. Cardiovascular disease involves thickening of the arteries (atherosclerosis), which interferes with the blood supply to organs and tissues, causing heart attacks and strokes. The two types of fats that can be measured in the blood are cholesterol and triglycerides. Cholesterol is measured as total cholesterol, and is considered to be abnormal if it is greater than 5.5 mmol/L. To complicate matters further, two fragments of cholesterol are usually measured: high-density lipoprotein (HDL cholesterol) and low-density lipoprotein (LDL cholesterol). It is believed that the LDL cholesterol is harmful, in that it causes thickening of the arteries, whereas the HDL cholesterol is protective and mops up other circulating fats. During the last decade community programmes have been instigated to encourage people to decrease their cholesterol levels by eating healthy diets and, where necessary, using cholesterol-lowering medications.

There has been a limited number of studies of the lipid profiles of women with polycystic ovaries or polycystic ovary syndrome. Although the studies that have been carried out report on a range of different comparisons, they seem to find consistently that there are poorer lipid profiles amongst women with polycystic ovary syndrome than amongst controls. An inconsistent relationship has been found between polycystic ovaries/polycystic ovary syndrome and lipid levels, although, overall, the findings are definitely negative. In particular, most of the studies have found lower levels of HDL (the 'good' or 'protective' form of cholesterol) in women with polycystic ovaries/polycystic ovary syndrome than amongst controls. Interestingly, one study found that these changes are more significant in women under the age of 40 years. As polycystic ovary syndrome becomes manifest during women's childbearing years, this gives further evidence to its effect on lipid metabolism.

There may be several reasons for the inconsistent findings of these studies. For example:

- most of the studies are very small,
- the reliability of a single measure of lipid fractions is poor, as these levels can vary markedly from day to day,
- no two of the studies have used the same definition of polycystic ovary syndrome for subjects and for controls and therefore the comparisons are always different,
- as body mass index (BMI) and lipid levels are closely related, the failure of these studies to take BMI fully into account leads to imprecision. As obesity and lipid levels are closely related, comparisons of women with and without polycystic ovary syndrome but with similar BMIs would help to clarify whether the differences in lipid levels are due to polycystic ovaries or to obesity.

Further information is therefore required before we can be certain about the effect of polycystic ovary syndrome on lipids, and whether being overweight (which many women with the condition are) is a significant contributing factor. However, the circumstantial evidence is that even having polycystic ovaries is likely to be a risk factor for lipid abnormalities.

Due to the definite association between abnormal lipids and increased cardiovascular risk, it would be sensible to screen women with polycystic ovaries or polycystic ovary syndrome for cholesterol and triglyceride levels. For those whose lipid levels are found to be abnormal, dietary and weight reduction measures should be strongly recommended in the first instance (see Chapter 7).

Cardiovascular disease

Recognized risk factors for cardiovascular disease include an increased waist:hip ratio, increased serum fats, high blood pressure and diabetes.

It has been known for about 20 years that elevated levels of cholesterol and abnormal lipids in the blood result in an increased risk of cardiovascular disease. In two large American studies it was clearly shown that death due to cardiovascular disease was closely related to raised levels of fats in the blood (raised triglycerides and reduced HDL cholesterol). The raised levels of insulin (hyperinsulinaemia) that are so common in women with polycystic ovary syndrome are now recognized to be responsible for a condition called metabolic syndrome. Metabolic syndrome is characterized by obesity (particularly increased fat deposition around the middle of the body, giving the apple shape), elevated levels of triglycerides (a type of fat that circulates in the body), raised cholesterol and insulin resistance. Both men and women who develop metabolic syndrome have an increased risk of developing high blood pressure and diabetes. Hypertension (high blood pressure) and diabetes have been found to be more common in women with polycystic ovary syndrome. Other studies have shown that even women with polycystic ovary syndrome who are not obese are at risk of hyperinsulinaemia and/or lipid abnormality, which suggests that they also have an increased risk of cardiovascular disease.

The Swedish study discussed above, which involved women who had had polycystic ovary syndrome diagnosed some 30 years previously, and followed them through until they reached 40-61 years of age, found that their risk of developing a myocardial infarction (heart attack) was seven times greater than that of the controls.

There are several reports in the literature showing a higher incidence of the risk factors of cardiovascular disease in women who have polycystic ovary syndrome. However, a large series from the UK involving women diagnosed with polycystic ovary syndrome between 1930 and 1979 did not show an increased mortality rate from cardiovascular disease compared to controls. Nevertheless, because disturbances of insulin resistance and lipid profiles are often associated with cardiovascular disease, and as disturbances of both lipids and carbohydrates are common in polycystic ovary syndrome, it is a small step to suggesting that the risk of cardiovascular disease is likely to be increased.

A possible relationship between lipid abnormalities and cardiovascular disease

From the evidence above, it may be concluded that women with polycystic ovary syndrome, especially those who are obese, have a higher risk of cardiovascular disease. Whether this actually results in more frequent hospital admissions or even deaths is still debatable.

A study in Auckland, New Zealand, looked at the incidence of polycystic ovaries amongst 143 women who required coronary angiography (examination of the blood vessels of the heart using a dye that shows up on x-ray) for previous chest pain or heart attack. It was found that women who had polycystic ovaries had more extensive disease than women who did not. In another study of women undergoing investigations of their coronary arteries, excessive hair growth and acne (possible signs of polycystic ovary syndrome) were twice as common in those with vessel disease as they were in those without it. A study of the vessels supplying blood to the brain (the carotid arteries) using ultrasound measurements of artery wall thickness found that thickening of these vessels (arteriosclerosis) was more common in women with polycystic ovary syndrome.

However, in 1998, the results were published of a large British study that followed 768 women with polycystic ovary syndrome diagnosed between 1930 and 1979. In this study, 59 women died as a result of ischaemic heart disease (disease of the coronary arteries leading to insufficient blood supply to the heart) - an incidence of heart disease that was no more frequent than would be expected in the general population.

Therefore, the suggestion that women with polycystic ovary syndrome (and thus less favourable lipid profiles and a higher incidence of diabetes) have a higher incidence of cardiovascular disease has not yet been proven.

One of the reasons why it is difficult to interpret the results of the studies published so far is that most of the women involved have been relatively young - the effect of atherosclerosis resulting in cardiovascular disease may become more apparent as women age. Further studies need to be carried out before any firm conclusions can be drawn.

High blood pressure

A similarly confounding factor is apparent when we look at the incidence of hypertension in women with polycystic ovary syndrome. Studies have reported high levels of both systolic and diastolic blood pressure in affected women when compared to controls, an effect that has been particularly apparent in the studies that have followed the women into their sixth decade. In a Swedish study, high blood pressure was found to be three times as common in women with polycystic ovary syndrome as it was in the controls. However, no adjustment has been made in these studies for BMI or other indices of obesity. Therefore, it is not clear whether the raised blood pressure reported is due to polycystic ovary syndrome alone or is related to obesity.

Is the cardiovascular risk of polycystic ovary syndrome a 'death hazard'?

The information discussed above certainly suggests that the markers for increased cardiovascular risk, such as unfavourable lipid changes, insulin resistance and possibly high blood pressure, are all more commonly present in women with polycystic ovary syndrome. It therefore seems reasonable to conclude that polycystic ovary syndrome is a health hazard; but is it a 'death hazard'? Do more women die because they have polycystic ovaries than would be expected? The only report of a study of mortality in relation to polycystic ovary status (the British study published in 1998) showed no increase in mortality rate. However, diabetes was mentioned as a possible contributory cause of death in almost four times as many women with polycystic ovary syndrome as in the controls.

Cancer

ENDOMETRIAL CANCER

It has long been recognized that unopposed oestrogens (i.e. oestrogen in the absence of associated progesterone) are an increased risk factor for cancer of the uterine lining (the endometrium). This can occur in women who do not ovulate regularly and therefore do not produce regular progesterone, or especially in the context of hormone replacement therapy (HRT) using oestrogen alone. Other risk factors include diabetes, obesity, hypertension and not having had children.

Hysterectomy for endometrial cancer may be more common in women with polycystic ovary syndrome. Endometrial cancer is uncommon in women under the age of 40, but in a Swedish study of women who developed it at a young age, symptoms of polycystic ovary syndrome, an increased BMI, increased hair growth and high blood pressure were far more common than normal. Also, a recent, large Israeli study involving nearly 2500 infertile women found a higher than expected incidence of endometrial carcinoma, as did a study from the Mayo Clinic in the USA. Again, there is, as yet, little understanding of whether it is polycystic ovary syndrome itself that is responsible for this increased risk or whether it is related to the associated factors of obesity and insulin resistance.

OVARIAN CANCER

The risk of ovarian cancer in women with polycystic ovary syndrome has been less studied than breast or uterine cancer and the data are conflicting. To complicate matters, women who take oral contraceptives are afforded significant protection against ovarian cancer and, as many women with polycystic ovaries are relatively infertile, fewer use oral contraceptives. There is one study on cancer and steroid hormones in the USA in which more women with ovarian cancer than controls self-reported that they had polycystic ovaries, with a risk ratio of 2.5:1. On the other hand, a large Danish study showed no association between ovarian cancer and a history of excess androgenic hormone secretion, which would be a marker for polycystic ovary syndrome.

BREAST CANCER

As far as breast cancer is concerned, there is no suggestion that women with polycystic ovary syndrome have any greater risk than the general population.

Conclusions

It is obvious that further studies need to be carried out to assess the long-term risks of polycystic ovary syndrome. These studies will have to be strict and uniform in their definition of polycystic ovaries and polycystic ovary syndrome. They will also have to be corrected for other risk factors such as obesity, treatment with hormones, and childbearing. The need to follow these women for several decades means that the results from prospective studies will not be available for many years. However, retrospective studies have the disadvantage of relying on past assessment of ovarian status.

S e v e n

Advice and lifestyle changes

The problems that predominate for women with polycystic ovary syndrome are many and varied. Some women require assistance with skin problems, if this is the predominant symptom during their teenage years, and some may need ovulation induction (see Chapter 10) when they wish to have children. Many women with polycystic ovary syndrome are overweight and need to be given advice about modifying their diet to control their weight and about lifestyle changes such as increasing the amount of exercise they take. Early intervention with lifestyle modifications may decrease the potential complications, as it has been suggested that women with polycystic ovary syndrome have a higher chance of developing diabetes and thickening of the walls of the arteries (atherosclerosis).

Body weight

It has long been recognized that certain clinical features of polycystic ovary syndrome improve when obese women lose weight. This applies to menstrual irregularity, acne and even hirsutism. It therefore seems logical that a programme of diet, exercise and lifestyle changes should be part of the management of women with polycystic ovary syndrome.

This is particularly relevant for women planning to become pregnant, as a high pre-pregnancy weight increases the risks of the pregnancy,

41

including those of high blood pressure, toxaemia, gestational diabetes and subsequent caesarian section. The risk of miscarriage is also increased in overweight women. Studies have shown that the dose of gonadotrophins required to induce ovulation (see page 76) increases with increasing body weight.

There is no consensus on the outcome of pregnancy with respect to body weight when women with polycystic ovary syndrome are treated by ovulation induction or in-vitro fertilization (IVF - see Chapters 10 and 12). It would appear that central obesity is the relevant factor for fertility. Simple obesity is associated with excess fat on the buttocks, whereas central obesity involves the deposition of fat around the abdomen, producing what is called the apple shape. Obesity associated with increased levels of male hormones is usually central obesity, and this is a recognized risk factor for cardiovascular disease.

STRATEGIES FOR WEIGHT LOSS

Appendix I (page 107) contains a table to calculate your body mass index. Chapter 8 explains the surgery that can be undertaken to reduce the weight of obese individuals who have not responded to the more conventional methods of weight loss.

Weight gain or weight loss can be compared to the petrol consumption of a motor car: the status of the fuel tank depends on the number of kilometres travelled and the amount of fuel used and replaced. With nutrition and weight gain or loss, the important formula is the number of kilojoules ingested minus the energy used up by activity. In order to lose weight, it is necessary either to decrease the kilojoules ingested by changing the amount and type of food eaten, or to increase the amount of energy used up by increasing exercise levels. It is best to do both: decrease the kilojoule intake and increase exercise.

People can also be compared to cars when it comes to consumption. Different people have different metabolic rates. This means that two people ingesting the same amount of kilojoules and undertaking the same amount of activity will not necessarily have the same weight loss or gain.

It is therefore important for individuals to adjust their energy intake and utilization in order to lose weight.

Other influences may also change our metabolism. For example, some hormones may increase weight gain, whereas others decrease it. Again, the car analogy can be used: someone who drives a car by putting his or her foot 'flat to the floor' and then slamming on the brakes will use more fuel per kilometre than someone who drives more carefully. It would appear that women with polycystic ovaries tend to put on weight, suggesting that they may be less efficient at using energy. How and why this happens are not fully understood, but the insulin resistance with higher insulin levels is probably responsible for sugars being taken up by cells and making them grow.

Only the principles of dieting are covered here; more specific advice can be obtained from a dietitian or from books written specifically for dieting.

When attempting to lose weight, it is important to consume a balanced diet. It is obvious that ingesting more kilojoules than are being used up by exercise will result in weight gain, and therefore the total amount of kilojoules consumed needs to be decreased. However, as well as decreasing the quantity of food eaten, attention should be paid to what is eaten: a diet that includes a wide variety of food types will ensure that all the nutrients, vitamins and minerals are obtained that are required by the body to maintain all its functions.

- Breads and cereals: these include bread, rolls, rice, pasta, cereals and biscuits.
- Fruit and vegetables: these are a source of carbohydrate, vitamin C, folate, fibre and iron.
- Meat and alternatives: these contain protein, niacin, vitamin B12, iron and zinc. Meat should be lean (with the fat removed); alternatives to meat are beans, lentils, and peas.
- Dairy foods: these include milk, cheese and yoghurt. Low-fat varieties should be eaten for weight reduction.

- Fats and oils: these contain essential fatty acids and fat-soluble vitamins A and D. The intake of these should be limited as they are high in energy. Polyunsaturated or mono-unsaturated fats are better than saturated fats such as butter, cream or lard.
- Fluids: it is important to drink plenty of fluids to supply the body's requirements. Fluids also help to distend the stomach and give a feeling of fullness. It is better not to include too many cups of tea or coffee as these contain caffeine, which is a diuretic and acts to excrete fluids from the body.

SOME HELPFUL BASIC PRINCIPLES FOR DIETING

- To lose weight, it is necessary to reduce fat intake.
- Gram for gram, fats contain more kilojoules than carbohydrates (more than twice as many) or proteins. Furthermore, once eaten, fats are less easily used up during exercise and are more likely to be deposited as fat stores on the abdominal wall, thighs, hips and arms. Also, fats do not give as much of a feeling of fullness as other food types, and therefore do not suppress appetite as efficiently.
- Many low-fat and reduced-fat foods are lower in fat than their equivalents but not necessarily *low* in fat. They therefore may still contain significant amounts of fat and thus too many kilojoules to allow weight loss. Nevertheless, a little fat is essential for good health, as it contains the fat-soluble vitamins mentioned above. It is suggested that no more than 25-30% of kilojoules per day should come from fats.
- It is also essential to eat sufficient fibre, which is contained in beans, grains, cereals, vegetables and fruits. Fibre also makes dieting easier, as it gives a feeling of being satisfied but contains few kilojoules; it also decreases the number of kilojoules absorbed from food.
- Sugars should also be reduced and taken in moderation. They should be taken in 'healthier' forms such as cereals, fruit juices, custard, flavoured milk, yoghurt and canned fruit, rather than in ice lollies, soft drinks, chocolates, cakes and pastries.

◆ Limiting alcohol consumption is an important part of dieting as alcoholic drinks can add significantly to the daily kilojoule intake. The rule should be no more than two standard drinks a day.

Lifestyle modification programmes

In the light of the above, a novel approach was developed in Adelaide with the setting up of a lifestyle modification group for overweight women with polycystic ovary syndrome. Although weight reduction is desirable, the basis of this treatment is not decreased calorie intake. The programme is comprehensive and includes a clear explanation of polycystic ovary syndrome. Individuals receive dietary advice and an exercise programme, and are also given peer group support.

It is recommended that the course be attended for 6 months and that the women's partners should be included. Meetings are held weekly and last for 2 hours, about half of which time is devoted to gentle exercises. The dietary advice is confined to healthy eating patterns and does not concentrate on drastic calorie reduction. Other lifestyle changes, such as stopping smoking and reducing alcohol intake, are also encouraged.

The Adelaide group has found that many of the women on this programme manage to achieve sustained weight loss. More than 90% have shown a dramatic improvement in their menstrual cycles. A significant number of spontaneous pregnancies has resulted, with a lower miscarriage rate than previously. Even women who are in an IVF programme for non-ovulation-related problems have shown an improvement in the outcome of their treatment.

This programme has shown clearly that an understanding of what the syndrome involves and some relatively straightforward modifications of lifestyle can have a significant impact on at least some of the symptoms of polycystic ovary syndrome. Similar programmes have been now been adopted elsewhere, with variable success.

E i g h t

Surgery for obesity

This chapter is a summary from a brochure produced by Mr Andrew Jamieson, a general surgeon specializing in obesity surgery.

Introduction

Surgical treatment to combat obesity follows the principle that the amounts of food and kilojoules that are absorbed in the bowel should be limited.

The stomach is the first part of the digestive system, and is the site where food that has been swallowed through the oesophagus is attacked by acids. It also acts as a reservoir for food (and can hold more than 1.5 litres), as the bowel can only cope with small amounts at a time.

When the stomach is full, a signal is transmitted back to the brain, which results in the person feeling full. As soon as the stomach contents are emptied into the bowel, the feeling of satisfaction disappears and is replaced by a feeling of hunger. If the messages from the stomach indicating hunger increase, the person will tend to eat more and will eventually become overweight.

Surgically assisted weight loss was first attempted in 1954 in the USA when a procedure was carried out to join a loop of bowel to bypass most of the small bowel, where nutrients are absorbed. Although the operation usually resulted in significant weight loss, it also had unfortunate side-effects such as diarrhoea, liver disease and kidney stones, which led to its abandonment.

In the 1960s, another procedure was developed in the USA, this time to bypass the stomach. Although this eliminated most of the side-effects of the small-bowel bypass operation, it was difficult to perform and had some associated long-term complications.

In the 1970s, a technique was introduced to shrink the size of the stomach by stapling - called gastroplasty. A variation of this technique, called gastric banding, has become popular since the 1980s and often achieves very good results. However, there can be technical problems with gastric banding, and further surgery may be needed.

Stomach stapling

The preferred method today involves forming a small pouch in the upper part of the stomach that effectively becomes the new, 'baby' stomach (Figure 8.1, page 48). The pouch is formed by a row of staples inserted longitudinally, leaving only a narrow opening between the pouch and the rest of the stomach. The amount of solid food that can fit into this new stomach at each meal is significantly reduced and a feeling of satisfaction occurs very quickly. This means that someone who has had stomach stapling feels full after eating only a small amount of solid food. This feeling of fullness lasts for several hours, until the stomach pouch empties. Therefore, the total daily intake of food is limited to three small, solid meals and the person does not feel hungry at any time. Thus, there is no temptation to gorge on other foods and increase the energy intake.

Before undergoing this major operation, which is a significant step to take, careful consideration should be given to its advantages and disadvantages. It should only be considered after more conservative measures such as supervised dieting have failed.

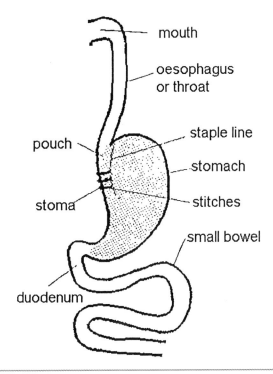

Figure 8.1 The changes to the stomach after stapling.

Surgical stapling does not in any way adversely affect fertility, but it would be wise not to try to conceive until weight reduction has been achieved. Fertility is more likely to return after weight has been lost, and there are significantly fewer complications of pregnancy for patients who have managed to lose weight.

SURGICAL PROCEDURE

The operation is performed in hospital and is quite a serious procedure. As it is difficult to give anaesthetics to people who are overweight, there is a significant anaesthetic risk associated with this operation. This risk is further compounded if the person is a smoker and

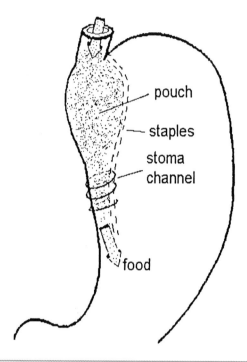

pouch

staples

stoma
channel

food

Figure 8.2 A new 'baby' stomach that results from stomach stapling.

therefore has an increased risk of breathing problems post-operatively and of wound pain caused by coughing. It is therefore important that people undergoing stomach stapling stop smoking for at least a month beforehand.

The operation can take up to about an hour to complete, depending on whether any technical difficulties are experienced. The abdomen is opened by an incision, about 10-15 cm long, which is made behind the ribs or down the middle of the body. If an abdominal scar is already present from a previous operation, the new incision may be made through it.

Once the stomach can be seen, a series of 33 staples is put through its wall to join the front and back walls together to form a new pouch. Stitches are put around the pouch to ensure it stays open but does not stretch (Figure 8.2, page 49).

POST-OPERATIVE RECOVERY

The operation usually involves a stay in hospital of a few days, during which time it is important for regular physiotherapy to be undertaken, with particular attention being paid to breathing and coughing exercises. It is also important for patients to get out of bed and move around as soon as possible after surgery to decrease the chance of blood clots (thromboses) forming in the legs.

The pain after this operation is not usually severe, and painkilling injections are not required for more than the first 24 hours, after which oral painkillers are normally sufficient.

No food must be eaten for the first day or two after the operation, and fluids are usually administered intravenously (i.e. through a tube inserted into a vein).

After discharge from hospital, patients are encouraged to be as active as possible, the limiting factor being any pain from the abdominal wound. As the staple line is within the abdominal wall, exercise will not affect it, although straining the stomach muscles will be painful. Anyone whose job involves heavy physical work or lifting will probably need to be off work for 4-6 weeks, but most people can usually return to work sooner than that.

EATING AFTER THE OPERATION

After the recovery phase, patients have to realize that they must alter their method of eating. Initially, only vitamin-enriched food is eaten and patients have to get used to feeling full after just a few teaspoons of semi-solid food. The capacity of the 'baby' pouch will increase over the first year or so and the amount that is needed to feel full will change. Although eating such small amounts may seem strange, remember that this is the aim of the procedure. Sufficient nutrition can be obtained by eating small amounts frequently.

After a few weeks, non-mashed solids can also be eaten, but these need to be chewed properly, with adequate lubrication. The important thing after undergoing this operation is not to eat to feel full, as the pouch is already full and putting excess food into it will just make you feel unwell. Once the pouch is filled up with solids, it is difficult to drink fluids, so these should be drunk before any solids are eaten. Also, fluids drunk at the same time as solids are being eaten will wash the food through the pouch, allowing too much to pass through, and therefore the appetite will not be satisfied and the operation will have been a waste of time.

Food should be eaten slowly and chewed properly, otherwise the pouch may overflow. The opening of the pouch is only 12 mm wide, and therefore nothing bigger than a pea should be swallowed. If solid food larger than this is eaten, it may become stuck in the pouch and cause abdominal pain and vomiting.

It is important to have a balanced diet, despite the small amounts of food that are being eaten, so that adequate vitamins and minerals are still absorbed.

SIDE-EFFECTS

Like most surgical procedures, stomach stapling can have some side-effects. The most significant of these is associated with the aim of the exercise - to restrict people to eating only small meals. If the advice given above is not followed, vomiting or regurgitation of food may occur; however, with care, there is usually no regurgitation at all. Indigestion (heartburn) - a burning feeling in the stomach going up into the chest - may result if too much food is eaten or if fluids are drunk with food. If this occurs, some of the stomach contents, including the acid, regurgitate into the oesophagus causing indigestion, which may be helped by taking antacids.

It is not unusual for patients who have undergone gastric stapling to experience constipation. Normal bowel movements consist mainly of fibre and, following this operation, the amount of fibre eaten is decreased. If constipation becomes a problem, more fluid should be consumed and fibre-containing foods, such as fruit and cereals, or liquid fibre preparations should be taken. Occasionally, patients may experience some dizziness if they stand up suddenly.

Some months after a successful operation, a significant amount of fat will have been lost and this sometimes leads to the problem of sagging, loose skin. If this does occur, it may be possible to undergo cosmetic surgery, such as a tummy tuck, to remove the excess skin. Exercise does help to some degree to prevent this looseness of skin developing.

COMPLICATIONS

As with most operations, complications can occur. These can be minor and hardly noticeable, or major. The risks of this operation for people without other medical complications are probably no greater than those of any other major surgical procedure. The most common complication is wound infection, which occurs in about 1 in 20 patients because of the amount of fatty tissue that has to be cut.

The most serious complication is inflammation of the lining of the abdominal cavity (peritonitis) that can result from leakage of stomach fluid. The other high-risk complication is the development of blood clots in the legs, which can pass in the blood vessels to the lungs (pulmonary embolism). To prevent this, anticoagulant drugs and the wearing of surgical stockings are usually prescribed. Both of these major complications occur in the first week or so after surgery.

The staples that are used in this operation are made of stainless steel or titanium, neither of which causes any long-term side-effects. They do not set off the metal detectors at airports and they do not rust or become dislodged and move to other sites in the body. The staples hold the walls of the stomach together for the first few post-operative weeks, after which healing occurs and the walls become naturally bound together.

Nine

Polycystic ovaries and the skin

Apart from menstrual irregularities, women with polycystic ovary syndrome most commonly seek medical intervention for skin problems, including increased hair growth (hirsutism) and acne. (Some women with polycystic ovary syndrome experience hair loss.) There is a marker of insulin resistance called acanthosis nigricans, characterized by increased keratin deposition and pigmentation, that is occasionally present in women with polycystic ovary syndrome who suffer from acne.

Acne

Acne is chronic inflammation of the sweat ducts of the skin. It usually occurs during the early teenage years and, although some acne lesions are common in all women, its severity varies. In most people it disappears by the age of 21, but it persists in the majority of women with polycystic ovary syndrome.

Due to the increased male hormone circulation associated with polycystic ovary syndrome, the sebaceous glands at the base of the hair follicles increase their secretions of sebum. As the androgens become more active, further enlargement of the sebaceous glands occurs and even more sebum is produced, which promotes the growth of a bacterium called *Propionibacterium acnes* (*P. acnes*), which thrives in the sebaceous environment. The bacterium digests the sebum, making it more viscous, as well as producing inflammatory by-products. In response to this inflammation, there is increased formation of the protein keratin, which plugs up the follicles, resulting in the development of small cysts called comedones, which are the initial lesions of acne. If these cysts are disrupted, they release inflammatory mediators, which results in the formation of a papule, pustule or cyst.

Acne primarily affects the face and, less often, the back and chest. It may present as blackheads (these are non-inflamed lesions with a black colour due to the laying down of the pigment melanin). When closed, these are known as whiteheads. The various lesions of acne often change from one type to another. They can result in scarring, which becomes significant in only a minority of people.

TREATMENT

Mild acne can be treated with topical creams that break down the keratin, such as azaleic acid or retinoids, or with antibiotics such as benzoyl peroxide, clindamycin lotion or erythromycin gel. In severe cases, antibiotics are often given orally; these antibiotics are usually of the tetracycline, erythromycin or trimethoprim group.

If antibiotic treatment fails, or the acne is significantly worse before menstrual periods, an anti-androgen is sometimes used. The two most common anti-androgens are spironolactone and cyproterone acetate. Some oral contraceptives aggravate acne and it is therefore important that an appropriate one is used, which, in general, will be one that is oestrogen dominant (i.e. with a relatively high oestrogen content). Biphasic pills are the most oestrogenic (Biphasil, Wyeth; Sequilar, Schering), followed by triphasic pills, but even better is the one containing progestogen in the form of cyproterone acetate (Diane 35, Schering), which provides progestogen in a form that not only has no male hormone activity, but also has definite anti-male hormone activity.

During the last decade, isotretinoin (Roaccutane) has become available. This drug belongs to a class of compounds called retinoids, which are derivatives of vitamin A. Its administration results in an 80% reduction of sebum excretion and, consequently, of *P. acnes* content within 4-8 weeks. Its precise mechanism of action is not yet understood, but its beneficial effect is probably due to its ability to decrease all major causative factors for acne: sebum production, comedogenesis (the production of comedones), skin bacterial content and inflammation. Its use results in long-term remission in more than 70% of cases. However, it has been linked to major fetal abnormalities of multiple systems and therefore adequate contraceptive measures (oral contraceptives of an oestrogen-dominant type to help the acne) need to be taken during treatment and for 1 month afterwards. A pregnancy test must be carried out before starting the medication.

Hirsutism

Hirsutism (or hairiness) is defined as hair growth in a woman resembling that of a man. The number of hair follicles usually remains constant, but their size and length increase, as does the pigmentation of the hair. As people of different races have different amounts of hair growth, it is often difficult to assess deviations from the norm. Although such deviations are sometimes perceived rather than real, they can result in anxiety and low self-esteem.

There are androgen receptors in the hair follicles and stimulating these increases the size of the hair produced by each follicle. The extent and severity of hirsutism are graded according to the system described by Ferriman and Galway (Figure 9.1, page 56). This grading system uses a score of 1 to 4 in each of nine hormonal sites, with a total score being derived by adding together the nine individual scores. It is therefore possible to assess changes in hair growth on a semi-quantitative scale by comparing progressive Ferriman-Galway scores.

TREATMENT
When assessing the outcome of any form of therapy, it has to be remembered that the hair follicles have a 3-month growth cycle, so no

Male-pattern hair growth in women

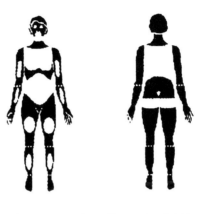

Demarcation of sights-anterior view   Demarcation of sights-posterior view

Figure 9.1 The Ferriman and Galway method of scoring hirsutism. (Reproduced by permission Cambridge University Press.)

improvement would be expected to be noticeable until treatment has been continuing for at least 3 months.

Cosmetic treatments The first line of treatment for increased hair growth involves the use of cosmetics, including bleaching, shaving, plucking, depilatory creams, electrolysis and laser. The use of peroxide bleach is often sufficient. In other situations, shaving may be all that is needed and, contrary to common belief, this does not affect the rate or duration of the growth of further hairs or the hair diameter. Plucking of hairs sometimes helps, and repeated attempts may lead to permanent hair follicle damage, resulting in finer hairs. However, this may cause inflammation, leading to increased pigmentation. Chemical depilatories usually contain thioglycates, which damage the hair shaft. The chemical is spread on the area and left for up to 15 minutes, after which it can be wiped away with the destroyed hairs. Unfortunately, skin irritation often results and this method is poorly tolerated in the armpit and on the face. Electrolysis (which involves passing an electric current down the hair follicle) is an approved method of permanent hair removal and results in the destruction of the root of the hair, known as the dermal papilla. The procedure is very operator dependent and can cause inflammation of the hair follicles, increased hair growth and scarring. There are various types of lasers that can be used to vaporize the target tissue. Several treatments are usually required for significant improvement, but none of the presently used lasers has been proved to destroy the hair permanently.

Weight loss Women who are overweight usually find their hirsutism improves with weight loss. This is associated with a rise in the concentration of sex hormone-binding globulin (SHBG), resulting in less circulating active testosterone.

Pharmacological agents Various pharmacological agents have been used in attempts to improve hair growth. As the hair growth cycle continues for several months, prolonged treatment is required before any improvement can be expected. Oral contraceptives may lead to some improvement by suppressing ovarian androgen production and increasing the levels of SHBG. An oestrogen-dominant pill or, preferably, one containing cyproterone acetate as the progestogen - such as Diane 35, which contains 2 mg in each daily dose - or a third-generation synthetic progestogen should be used. Third-generation progestogens have been developed during the last decade, and these have superseded the first-generation progestogens that were developed in the 1960s and the second-generation progestogens developed in the 1970s. Each refinement in progestogen has resulted in a reduction in the male hormone-type side-effects.

Cyproterone acetate (the hormone in Diane 35, see above), although having a progesterone-like effect on the lining of the womb, is a specific androgen antagonist. When administered in an oral contraceptive pill, it is given as a small dose (2 mg) every day. If a stronger effect is required, it is given with cyclic oestrogen and is used for 10 days each month at a dose of 50-100 mg. Its side-effects include loss of sex drive, some weight gain, fatigue, breast tenderness and gastrointestinal upsets as well as headache and depressed mood.

Another chemical treatment involves the use of an oral diuretic (a 'water tablet') called spironolactone. This reduces the availability of active testosterone by interfering with its production and accelerating its clearance from the body. The usual dose is 100-200 mg per day and the potential side-effects include menstrual irregularities, breast tenderness, stomach upsets, headaches and dizziness. As spironolactone also increases the potassium concentration in the body, which can have serious side-effects, the blood level of potassium needs to be checked regularly during treatment.

Another hormone that can be used is flutamide, which is a non-steroidal anti-androgen. It works by blocking the androgen receptors and preventing testosterone attaching to them. Its side-effects include dry skin, menstrual disturbance, fatigue, decreased sex drive and gastric upsets.

Androgenic alopecia

This condition involves progressive, non-scarring scalp hair loss. It usually occurs because of an inherited disposition and the increased circulation of the male hormones associated with polycystic ovary syndrome. It is common in women in their twenties to forties. The usual pattern of hair loss is diffused over the crown, with preservation of the frontal hairline associated with widening of the parting.

TREATMENT

Some studies have shown that weight loss is of benefit in androgenic alopecia, and the use of camouflage with appropriate hair styling may be all that is required.

Minoxidil is a medication that inhibits hair loss and can be used as a topical lotion applied in a 2% or 5% solution. It is massaged into the scalp and applied to both bald and vulnerable areas. Several months of treatment are needed before any change is noticed. The side-effects of minoxidil include redness and itching as well as a dry scalp.

Cyproterone and spironolactone have been used for the treatment of androgenic alopecia in doses similar to those used for hirsutism. Usually, a 3-6-month course of treatment is required before any change becomes apparent.

A major problem of assessing the effect of treatment is that the goal is the arrest of any further hair loss, with regrowth of hair being a welcome, but less likely, outcome. Photographs are sometimes taken in an attempt to assess any changes objectively, but even then the interpretation of clinical photographs is difficult. The recent introduction of digital clinical photography with stereotactic stabilizing devices has at least improved the accuracy of assessing treatment response.

Acanthosis nigricans

This is an eruption of skin, with increased keratin, papillomatosis (giving the skin a velvety appearance) and pigmentation. It usually occurs in the armpits, but may also arise in the nape of the neck and under the breasts. Almost all the women who develop this condition have polycystic ovaries and almost all are insulin resistant.

Ten

Ovulation induction

Even without treatment, many women with polycystic ovary syndrome will conceive spontaneously, but those who do not do so may wish to consider ovulation induction. Before making a decision about this treatment, there are some factors that need to be assessed. (Appendix IV contains some commonly asked questions concerning ovulation induction, and their answers.)

Pre-treatment considerations

MENSTRUATION

In the most severe cases, women experience a total lack of menstruation (amenorrhoea). If this resolves spontaneously, ovulation will precede menstruation. It is possible for women to conceive without menstruating, which is simply the sloughing off of the endometrium in preparation for the development of the next crop of ovarian follicles. Therefore, some women may conceive without having had a period, and they may not realize they are pregnant until well into the pregnancy.

Women with irregular periods also usually ovulate irregularly. There is some suggestion that ovulation that occurs every 6-12 weeks results in the production of less-fertile oocytes than those produced when ovulation is regular. A woman who ovulates every 8-12 weeks might have four to six chances a year of conceiving, compared to the 13 chances of someone who ovulates every 4 weeks.

The principle of treatment for all women who wish to become pregnant is to try to restore regular, monthly ovulation and menstruation.

OBESITY

Another factor that needs to be considered prior to inducing ovulation is that of lifestyle changes. These are discussed in more detail in Chapter 7, but the principal aim should be to encourage weight loss prior to conceiving in women with polycystic ovary syndrome who are obese. Even moderate obesity will inhibit ovulation and many women with polycystic ovary syndrome return to spontaneous, regular ovulation if they lose some body weight and get back to what is considered a normal body mass index (BMI). The BMI is a formula derived by calculating the weight of the woman in kilograms divided by her height in metres squared (see Appendix I), i.e.

$$BMI = \frac{weight \; (kg)}{height \; x \; height \; (m^2)}$$

A normal BMI is 21-26; women who are underweight have a BMI of less than 21 and women who are overweight have a BMI of 27 or greater (see Appendix I). It is not unusual for women with polycystic ovary syndrome and absence of ovulation (anovulation) to have a BMI in the high 30s.

Another interesting finding in women with polycystic ovary syndrome is that their body fat distribution changes. When the waist and hip circumferences are measured, it is the waist circumference that is greater than normal (see Chapter 7). Unfortunately, achieving weight reduction is difficult for everybody, but even more so for women with polycystic ovaries. For some reason their metabolic status conspires against weight loss and this is why educational, weight loss and exercise classes have been instituted for obese women with polycystic ovary syndrome, with such names as 'The Big Girls' Groups' (see Chapter 7).

Being overweight is a real handicap for ovulation induction. The veins are usually hard to locate and therefore blood tests are more stressful and difficult, and ovarian scanning is more complicated due to the increased fatty tissue. Of course, pregnancy also carries a greater risk in overweight women, with a higher risk of miscarriage, an increased chance of developing diabetes of pregnancy (gestational diabetes), high blood pressure and problems with delivery. All these potential problems are extra incentives to try to lose weight.

The physiology of ovulation

This is discussed in detail in Chapter 2, and is only summarized here. The aim of ovulation induction for women who do not ovulate is to mimic the natural process and to normalize the functions of the hypothalamus, pituitary gland and ovary.

Before explaining the use of ovulation induction for women who are anovulatory, it is important to understand the physiology of ovulation.

Ovulation is controlled by the pituitary gland in the brain. This gland is the size of a cherry and is located behind the bridge of the nose. It is controlled by the hypothalamus, which is in the central part of the brain, just above the pituitary gland (Figure 10.1, page 63). As well as being the central computer for ovulation, the pituitary gland is also involved with the secretion of hormones, including growth hormone and hormones stimulating the thyroid gland (in the neck) and adrenal glands (above the kidneys). The first hormone to consider is follicle-stimulating hormone (FSH). As its name implies, this hormone is pivotal in stimulating the unripe follicles within the ovary to develop into ripe follicles. The FSH level is elevated in the first few days of the menstrual cycle and this triggers the development of a group of follicles (Figure 10.2, page 63). In the natural situation, one of the developing follicles is destined to ovulate and become the 'leading follicle'. In humans, this follicle has the ability to suppress the other developing follicles so that, usually, in a natural, spontaneous cycle, only one follicle matures and ovulates. This

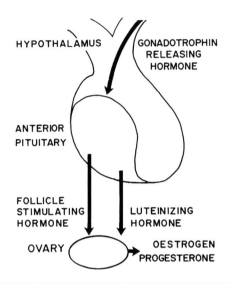

Figure 10.1 The interaction of the hypothalamus, pituitary gland and ovary.

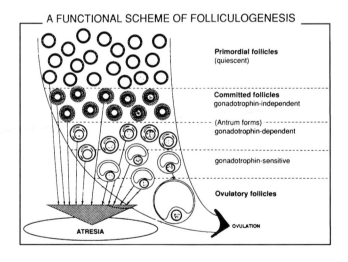

Figure 10.2 How a crop of follicles starts to grow, resulting in one dominant follicle.

process does not occur in animals, which is why humans tend to produce a single fetus, whereas animals have litters.

As mentioned in Chapter 2, as the leading follicle develops, it is like a growing hen's egg on the surface of the ovary. The ovum is equivalent to the egg yolk and will subsequently become fertilized and divide to form the embryo. The egg white and the eggshell surround the ovum. The egg white contains cells called granulosa cells, which are responsible for secreting the hormone oestrogen. Oestrogen acts on the pituitary gland and the hypothalamus and has a negative effect on the production of FSH. This process is not dissimilar to that of a thermostat in the heating system that turns off the boiler when an adequate temperature is reached. The secreted oestrogen 'turns off' the FSH so that only enough is produced to stimulate the growth of one batch of follicles with a single leading follicle.

Once the follicle is mature, a second hormone, luteinizing hormone (LH), is secreted. LH is usually secreted at basal levels (less than 10 international units (IU) per mL) throughout the menstrual cycle, but, for the 24 hours prior to ovulation, there is a very sharp peak (which can be up to 100 IU per mL). Ovulation occurs about 24 hours after the peak of LH secretion. As with many medical terms, the name luteinizing hormone comes from Latin, although it might be better termed 'ovulating hormone' as it is this hormone that causes ovulation.

Ovulation involves the mature egg coming to the surface of the ovary. LH is responsible for the cracking of the 'shell' and the release of the ovum, which subsequently passes down the fallopian tube. The cells in the egg white and the egg shell stay behind on the ovary and secrete both oestrogen and progesterone, developing a yellow appearance and forming the corpus luteum. In Latin, corpus luteum means yellow body, and it is the induction of this 'luteinization' that gives LH its name.

The hormones secreted by the developing follicle and the corpus luteum are essential in priming the female body for conception. The oestrogen secreted during the first phase of the growth of the follicle is responsible for the thickening of the lining of the uterus (the endometrium) and for inducing the fertile cervical mucus, which is copious, clear and elastic. The combined oestrogen and progesterone are also responsible for the nutrient content of the endometrium and for providing a suitable environment in which the embryo can develop.

The corpus luteum has a life of only 10-14 days and, therefore, if conception does not occur within this time, the oestrogen and progesterone levels drop and the lining of the uterus is sloughed off. This results in menstruation.

If conception has occurred, the early embryo secretes a hormone called beta human chorionic gonadotrophin (ßHCG). The presence of this hormone stimulates the corpus luteum to continue to function and it is the ßHCG in the blood that is detected when a pregnancy test is performed for early conception. The levels within the blood are measurable by the time the next menstrual period is missed - about 14 days after ovulation.

Reasons for seeking ovulation induction

Unless a woman has consulted a dermatologist because of acne or increased hair growth during her teenage years, or has been seen by a gynaecologist for irregular menstruation prior to starting to take a contraceptive pill, she may seek medical help for the first time when she fails to conceive. In many cases, women have irregular periods after discontinuing oral contraception and find that no pregnancy occurs after some months of unprotected intercourse. They usually consult their family doctor, who may do some blood tests and refer them to a gynaecologist because of abnormal ovulation.

Tests and useful information

MEDICAL HISTORY
For the clinical treatment of lack of ovulation - ovulation induction - the diagnosis of polycystic ovaries is not essential. However, to optimize

treatment and minimize the risk of being overstimulated, it is useful to know what the ovaries look like. An astute gynaecologist will obtain details of the woman's medical history, including:

- the age she started menstruating,
- whether her periods were initially regular,
- if she was previously taking oral contraceptives, whether menstruation re-commenced after she stopped,
- the frequency of menstruation, i.e. the length of time from the start of one period to the start of the next,
- the number of days each menstrual period lasts.

Other useful information includes details of possible symptoms associated with anovulation, such as increased hair growth, the presence of acne, and episodes of weight gain or weight loss.

Any relevant general medical history should also be recorded, including:

- any serious medical diseases, particularly hormone-related problems such as thyroid disease or diabetes,
- any medications that are being taken that might interfere with ovulation,
- previous operations that could jeopardise the tubes,
- the regularity and adequacy of sexual intercourse.

PHYSICAL AND VAGINAL EXAMINATIONS

A physical examination is usually required, and a note is taken of whether breast development is normal and whether there is increased hair growth. A vaginal examination is usually done to determine the size, shape and position of the uterus, and to palpate the ovaries for any enlargement. Polycystic ovaries are usually not palpable on a routine vaginal examination. A cervical smear test should also be performed if this has not been done recently.

BASELINE INVESTIGATIONS

Numerous baseline investigations are usually carried out before treatment is commenced. These include confirming that the woman is immune to German measles (rubella) and measuring the levels of the hormones involved in the control of the ovaries - FSH, LH, oestrogen and progesterone. The level of the hormone prolactin is also measured because elevated levels of this hormone can cause anovulation in some women (see below). Often, if polycystic ovary syndrome is suspected, the blood levels of the male-type hormones testosterone, dehydroepiandrosterone and sex hormone-binding globulin (SHBG) are also measured. It is now becoming common practice to measure the lipids in the blood and also glucose tolerance to unmask the presence of a diabetic tendency.

It must also be remembered that it 'takes two to tango' and, before starting a woman on fertility treatment, her partner's semen should also be analysed (see Appendix II).

Occasionally, a condition called premature menopause is diagnosed. This is usually associated with the total absence of periods and significantly elevated levels of FSH. These factors indicate that there are no follicles left in the ovary that are able to respond and therefore ovulation induction would not be successful. The possibility of ovum donation would then need to be considered.

Before ovulation induction is commenced, a baseline ultrasound examination (see page 19) should be performed to confirm whether polycystic ovaries are present and to look for any ovarian pathology.

RAISED PROLACTIN LEVELS

Another cause of anovulation that needs to be diagnosed before treatment is commenced is a raised level of the hormone prolactin. Prolactin is made by the pituitary gland and is involved in breast-feeding. However, even women who are not pregnant may sometimes have elevated prolactin levels, which can result in the cessation of ovulation. If the prolactin level is significantly elevated (more than four times the upper limits of normal), an investigation of the pituitary gland for the presence of a tumour should be undertaken using a computerized axial tomography (CAT) scan. If the prolactin level is only mildly elevated, it can be normalized by treatment with hormones without the need for any further investigations.

The first line of treatment for an elevated prolactin level is an oral medication to suppress it (Figure 10.3, page 69). One such option is bromocriptine, which is taken orally on a daily basis, starting off as a small dose and building up until the prolactin level has returned to normal. The disadvantage of bromocriptine is that it causes some nausea, although it is usually well tolerated if gradually built up from a low dose. Bromocriptine should be administered in the evening and at meal times so that any nausea occurs during sleep.

The other option is to use a twice-weekly medication of cabergoline and, again, build the dose up gradually until the prolactin level is normalized. For some women, even when the prolactin level returns to normal, ovulation does not recur and other methods of ovulation induction need to be used as well.

Clomiphene citrate

Most women, especially those with polycystic ovaries, have prolactin and FSH levels within the normal range and are therefore candidates for ovulation induction with oral medication, usually clomiphene citrate, which is a chemical with a structure very similar to that of oestrogen.

Clomiphene citrate acts by blocking the oestrogen receptors in the hypothalamus and pituitary, which respond as they would if not enough FSH had been produced (rather like covering up the thermostat of a central heating system so that it does not register the rising temperature). Consequently, FSH continues to be secreted in an attempt to prime the ovary (Figure 10.4, page 69).

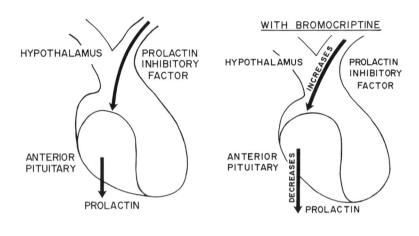

Figure 10.3 The management of raised prolactin.

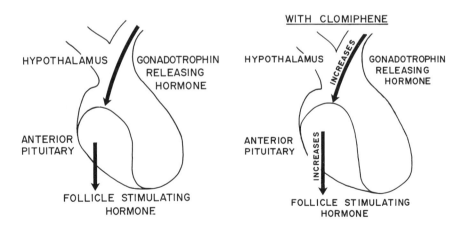

Figure 10.4 The effect of clomiphene on the pituitary gland and the response of FSH.

A 50-mg tablet of clomiphene citrate is taken daily for 5 days during the early part of the menstrual cycle. As women with polycystic ovary syndrome often do not have regular cycles, it may be several weeks before they can start on treatment with clomiphene citrate. For these women, a menstrual period can sometimes be induced if progestogen tablets are taken for 5-10 days. When the progestogen tablets are stopped, the endometrium comes away, which results in a 'withdrawal bleed'. The first day of bleeding is then documented as the first day of the menstrual cycle.

There are various ways of administering clomiphene citrate. Some doctors prescribe it from the second to the sixth day of the cycle, others from the fifth to the ninth day. The starting dose for women with polycystic ovary syndrome who are experiencing some menstruation should be 25 mg a day for 5 days. They therefore need to break their (50 mg) tablets in half: it does not matter if the two halves are not exactly the same size, as the remaining dose will be taken the following day. All the tablets should be taken at about the same time each day, which can be in the morning, at midday or in the evening.

The response to clomiphene citrate is best assessed in two ways.

1. A *temperature chart* is very useful (Figure 10.5, page 71). This will not only record the days of intercourse, but will also give a 'guestimate' of the time of ovulation. The elevation of the temperature during the second half of the cycle will also give some indication of how efficient the ovulation has been.
2. A *blood test* is a useful adjunct to the temperature chart. Blood should be taken around day 21 of the cycle, give or take a couple of days, and the oestrogen and progesterone levels measured. The level of oestrogen secreted will give some indication of the function of the ovaries and whether one or more follicles have developed. A raised progesterone level is circumstantial evidence that ovulation has taken place.

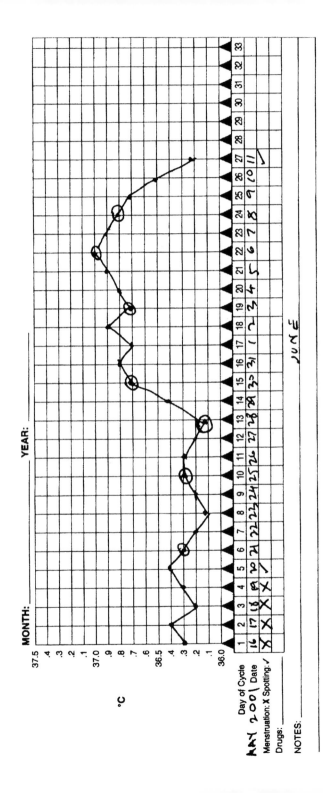

Figure 10.5 An ovulatory temperature chart. Note the elevation in the second half of the chart due to ovulation and progesterone secretion, with a small dip at ovulation on day 14. (This is a biphasic chart as it is elevated in the second half and has two phases.)

71

In addition, some reproductive gynaecologists follow the woman's response by using transvaginal ultrasound to look at the follicular development on the ovary. Although this does aid the assessment of a problematic patient, it involves extra inconvenience, discomfort and cost that are not absolutely essential.

The best-case scenario as a response to the first course of clomiphene citrate is for ovulation to take place around day 10-14 of the cycle, for intercourse to take place at the appropriate time, and subsequently for there to be an elevation in the temperature chart and for ovulatory levels of both oestrogen and progesterone to be found when a blood test is done at day 21. The perfect scenario is for the temperature chart to remain elevated (Figure 10.6, page 73), for there to be no subsequent menstrual period, and for the woman to have conceived during her first cycle. This happens in about 20% of women with polycystic ovaries being treated with clomiphene citrate.

If a pregnancy has occurred, no further intervention is necessary. However, a pregnancy test should be done to confirm that conception has occurred, and an ultrasound examination at 6-7 weeks of gestation is recommended to confirm the viability of the pregnancy and to determine whether more than one oocyte was ovulated, with the possibility of a multiple pregnancy. With the regime of clomiphene citrate suggested above, the chances of a multiple pregnancy are well under 5%.

The second best-case scenario is for ovulation to have taken place and for spontaneous menstruation to occur at about day 28-32 of the menstrual cycle.

If ovulation has occurred by day 16 of the treatment cycle but conception has not, the same dose of clomiphene citrate should be used for the next cycle. If the cycle does not result in ovulation, or if ovulation was delayed beyond about day 17, the dose of clomiphene citrate for the next ovulation induction cycle should be increased from 25 mg to 50 mg a day, again administered for the same 5 days.

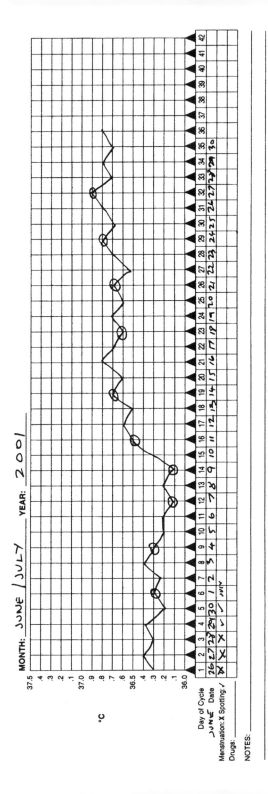

Figure 10.6 A temperature chart showing conception. Note the temperature remains elevated in the second phase due to the persistent secretion of progesterone by the early pregnancy, and there is no menstrual period.

73

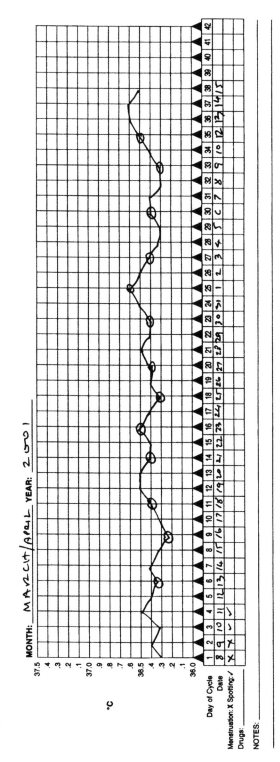

74

Figure 10.7 A monophasic temperature chart showing no ovulation. As there is no ovulation, no progesterone has been produced and the temperature does not rise.

If there has been no response, as judged by a lack of elevation on the temperature chart (Figure 10.7, page 74), no rise in the level of progesterone and an insignificant rise in the oestrogen level, it is unlikely that a menstrual period will result. It may then be necessary to induce another menstrual period by administering progestogen tablets for 5-10 days.

Progestogen administration that does not result in a withdrawal bleed is a very poor prognostic sign. It means that the woman is very unlikely to respond to ovulation induction by simple oral agents. The same treatment regime as that described above should then be followed, with progressively higher doses of clomiphene citrate, until satisfactory ovulation is achieved or a maximal dose of 150 mg per day (three tablets) has been reached. If satisfactory ovulation is achieved, the same dose of clomiphene citrate should be administered in subsequent cycles.

It is recommended that three ovulations should be induced in a woman who has no other obvious cause for her subfertility. If pregnancy does not occur after three ovulations have been confirmed, in association with well-timed intercourse with a fertile male partner, it is imperative to look for other factors explaining the subfertility. This would necessitate a diagnostic laparoscopy (see page 84) with dye studies of the fallopian tubes. It is also important to confirm that the semen analysis is satisfactory.

If conception occurs in any of the clomiphene citrate cycles, the routine discussed above should be followed. The level of serum ßHCG should be measured to confirm the pregnancy, and a vaginal ultrasound should be carried out at 6-7 weeks to confirm viability and the number of gestation sacs. Women with polycystic ovary syndrome have a higher risk of spontaneous miscarriage, and a repeat scan at 10-12 weeks is recommended.

Alternative treatments

There are a number of other options for women who fail to conceive with clomiphene citrate.

It has already been mentioned that polycystic ovary syndrome is frequently associated with a condition called insulin resistance, in which women need higher levels of insulin to keep their blood-sugar levels normal. There are a number of oral agents available that can counteract this insulin resistance and these are used for the treatment of diabetics, especially those who develop this condition later in life.

METFORMIN

Most of the work done in this field in relation to women with polycystic ovary syndrome has involved the use of the oral anti-diabetic medication metformin. There is some suggestion that women who do not respond to clomiphene citrate may become responsive to it after treatment with a combination of clomiphene and metformin, subsequently ovulating and becoming pregnant. Although the early reports from the USA are promising, there need to be some large-scale, controlled studies to confirm the value of the treatment. Nevertheless, it would be reasonable to try this for a few months before proceeding to further treatment. The side-effects of metformin therapy are diarrhoea and flatulence.

GLITAZONES

Some new medications - the glitazones, which counteract insulin resistance - are now being used for diabetics, and are being investigated as a possible way of counteracting insulin resistance in polycystic ovary syndrome. Whether these medications play any role in preventing the long-term complications has not yet been evaluated. If insulin resistance is the basic metabolic problem in polycystic ovary syndrome, counteracting this should 'control' the disease. However, we do not have any evidence for this yet, and long-term studies need to be carried out before these medications should be prescribed.

GONADOTROPHIN INJECTIONS

There are two further options for women who fail to ovulate following treatment with clomiphene citrate: a surgical approach and the use of ovulation induction injections. The surgical treatment of polycystic ovary syndrome is considered in the next chapter; the medical treatment is discussed in detail below.

As there is a significant risk of overstimulating the ovary, resulting in multiple pregnancies and/or a condition called ovarian hyperstimulation syndrome (see page 81), the supervision of ovulation induction with gonadotrophins is a highly skilled procedure and is usually undertaken by clinicians specializing in reproductive gynaecology. The treatment has been available for many years.

Because treatment with injections is expensive and far more time consuming and invasive than that with oral tablets, it is recommended that women have a diagnostic laparoscopy (see page 84) to rule out any other cause for their subfertility before embarking on ovulation induction with gonadotrophins.

Gonadotrophins are hormones that contain FSH. Rather than trying to stimulate the woman's own production of FSH and the maturation of follicles in her ovary, this treatment involves administering the FSH by injection on a daily basis; it thus acts directly on the woman's ovary rather than through the hypothalamo-pituitary route.

Treatment involves either waiting for a spontaneous period or inducing a withdrawal bleed, as discussed above for progestogen. Within the first 2 days of the menstrual cycle, a low dose of FSH is administered (50-75 units per day). The response is assessed by measuring the oestrogen level in the blood to see how the ovarian follicles are functioning and/or by transvaginal ultrasound imaging of the ovaries to assess the number and size of any follicles. Routine treatment would require this to be performed twice a week.

If there is no response, as judged by a rise in oestrogen levels or growth of ovarian follicles (on ultrasound) within 7-10 days, the dose of FSH is gradually increased. The aim is to produce two or three mature follicles only. If more follicles are produced and all ovulate, a multiple pregnancy may occur. The ovaries of women with polycystic ovary syndrome are very prone to over-reacting and suddenly producing a larger number of follicles. If this does occur, the ovulation of these follicles should not be triggered and the cycle should be abandoned, the couple being advised not to have intercourse because follicles can spontaneously still ovulate on their own without the ovulatory hormone being administered.

In a cycle with an ideal response, two or three follicles will mature together. When they reach the size of about 16-18 mm in diameter, as measured by transvaginal ultrasound (these follicles usually grow about 2 mm per day), ovulation can be triggered. Natural ovulation is stimulated by the woman's own LH, but, for ovulation induction, a hormone has to be used that is chemically very similar to LH - HCG, the early pregnancy hormone. This hormone is purified from the excretions of pregnant women and used for injection. The same recombinant DNA technology that enables the production of FSH has also been utilized to produce LH. Recombinant LH is currently undergoing clinical trials and should be available for clinical use within the next few years.

Once the HCG injection has been administered, in a single dose of 3000-5000 IU, ovulation usually occurs 24-36 hours later. The woman and her partner are asked to have intercourse over the next couple of days and the response is monitored by the measurement of the oestrogen and progesterone levels in the woman's blood over the next week or two. Because the cycle is artificial, it is believed that the function of the corpus luteum needs to be aided by booster doses of HCG. These doses are usually administered about three times at approximately 3-day intervals. If the woman has adequate levels of progesterone after ovulation, it is not considered necessary to administer the booster doses of HCG. This decision is made on a case by case, day by day basis by the clinician managing the woman's ovulation induction.

Complications of treatment The first complication may be that the woman does not respond to the treatment. In the absence of a raised FSH level, most women will respond to gonadotrophins given the appropriate dose. As the dose of gonadotrophin is increased in a stepwise fashion at 7-10-day intervals, it is possible that several weeks of injections may be required in order to achieve a response.

Another possible disappointment may be that, although the woman responds and does make some follicles, ovulation does not occur. If this happens, despite appropriate growth of follicles as determined by ultrasound, a higher dose of HCG is used in subsequent cycles to trigger ovulation.

It is also possible for ovulation to occur but for there to be no subsequent pregnancy. Most women would be expected to conceive within three to six confirmed ovulations. If a pregnancy still does not occur, some other infertility factor should be suspected and it may be necessary to consider in-vitro fertilization (see Chapter 12).

Another potential complication is that the woman may respond too well, several follicles being ovulated and a multiple pregnancy resulting. The cut-off point in most clinics is for ovulation to be induced as long as there are no more than three pre-ovulatory-sized follicles, which should mean that 80% of the pregnancies are singleton. An accepted multiple pregnancy rate is 20%; most are twins, with only occasionally triplets. Unfortunately, women can sometimes react in unusual ways. Although there may only be three pre-ovulatory-sized follicles, some smaller follicles may also ovulate and result in high-multiple pregnancies. Fortunately, up to a quarter of multiple pregnancies that are detected on the first ultrasound reduce spontaneously, i.e. not all of the embryos continue to grow.

Sources of gonadotrophins There were two initial sources of FSH: urinary gonadotrophins from the urine of post-menopausal women, which resulted in the first pregnancy in 1962, and pituitary gonadotrophins, which were used in Australia from 1967 to 1985. Although the treatment resulted in many women being able to conceive who otherwise would not have been able to do so, the association of pituitary gonadotrophins with a virus-like (prion) infection resulting in Creutzfeld-Jakob disease (CJD) has caused them to be abandoned.

CJD is a generative disease of the brain caused by a very small prion. Infection with this prion leads to premature dementia and subsequent death. Unfortunately, there is no method available to test for the presence of this prion in tissues such as blood or nervous tissue, even in people who are infected. The harmful effects of the infection do not become manifest for as long as 10-15 years. The infection has been known to have been transmitted to patients after infected patients have undergone operations on the brain, but other modes of transmission are not understood. In order to obtain FSH in the 1960s, pituitary glands were collected at post-mortem examinations and two hormone preparations were extracted from them, concentrated and purified. One of these hormones was growth hormone, which was used to treat children who were not growing at a normal rate and which prevented short stature. The other was human pituitary gonadotrophin (HPG), which was a combination of FSH and LH. In Australia, the use of HPG was made available free of charge for use in ovulation induction by the Department of Health. As soon as the association between CJD and HPG became apparent in April 1985, the use of HPG to induce ovulation was stopped. Fortunately, of the 1544 women treated over an 18-year period in Australia, only five appear to have been infected with the virus.

Urinary gonadotrophins were also used as a source of FSH for ovulation induction. Because women past their reproductive years cannot mature ovarian follicles, they have low levels of oestrogen, with a consequent rise in FSH levels in their blood. This FSH is excreted in their urine, which can be collected and the gonadotrophins extracted, concentrated and purified. Urinary gonadotrophins were the only source of FSH from the mid-1980s until the late 1990s. No similar problems of the transmission of any recognized infective material have been experienced with urinary gonadotrophins. However, although they have undergone a number of refinements during the last 40 years, they are now also obsolete.

FSH is now obtained by recombinant DNA technology, in which the hormone is synthesized in the laboratory. This has a number of advantages:

- it avoids the need to use hormones obtained from human tissue,
- it ensures that there is the same dose in every ampoule prepared and supplies are unlimited,

- it can be administered by injecting into the fatty tissue under the skin rather than into muscle.

Its only disadvantage is that it is more expensive. Fortunately, in Australia, in appropriate cases the cost is covered under the Pharmaceutical Benefits Scheme, but its use in each country will have to be assessed on a cost-benefit basis.

To answer the questions that women commonly ask before and during ovulation induction with injections of FSH, the Monash Ovulation Induction Service has produced a question and answer booklet. This is reproduced in a modified form in Appendix IV.

Fetal reduction

If a multiple pregnancy does continue and the woman feels she does not want to undergo the increased risk involved, a procedure called fetal reduction is sometimes performed. This involves the injection of potassium chloride into one or more embryos at 8-10 weeks of gestation. Some couples do not find this morally acceptable, and there is the risk of losing all the fetuses if the pregnancy continues without intervention. There is not a great deal of experience of fetal reduction in Australia, but results of studies from other countries suggest that, in 10-20% of cases, all the embryos will be lost. The acceptability as well as the risks and benefits of fetal reduction should be discussed with the clinician who is supervising the pregnancy.

Ovarian hyperstimulation syndrome

In very rare cases, several follicles may develop on the ovary, resulting in it becoming large, sore and swollen. This is associated with disturbance of the woman's fluid balance, with increased fluid accumulating in the peritoneal cavity of the abdomen and even in the lungs, which can make breathing difficult and also predisposes to coagulation of blood within the blood vessels - known as a thrombosis.

Occasionally, women are so unwell that they have to be hospitalized and given anticoagulants and pain relief. There have been very rare, but occasional, cases of fatal complications of thrombosis of the brain or lungs. Although this complication is far more common in women undergoing in-vitro fertilization than ovulation induction, the possibility of it occurring does have to be borne in mind. (See Chapter 12 for a more detailed explanation of this syndrome.)

Why not proceed with multiple pregnancies?

Whereas, for a subfertile couple, it may seem ideal to have two or three babies after only one pregnancy, and therefore for the family to be complete with a multiple pregnancy, even giving birth to twins - but particularly to triplets - is far more risky than giving birth to one child.

The chance of the babies failing to survive the birth is twice as high for twins and three times as high for triplets. Even if they are delivered alive, there is an increased risk of cerebral palsy - a condition involving a degree of brain injury during or prior to birth that results in the child's physical or mental functioning being compromised. The risk of cerebral palsy is up to five times higher for twins and possibly up to 20 times higher for triplets compared to singletons.

Prematurity is also more common with multiple pregnancies, and this is partly the cause of the subsequent complications. Even if the children are born healthy, there are significant long-term medical and social implications, including learning disability, language delays, attention behavioural problems and increased divorce rate amongst parents. There is, of course, also increased stress for the parents during the first few years of parenting.

Eleven

Surgical treatment to induce ovulation

The history of surgical treatment

As discussed in Chapter 1, the specialty of reproductive gynaecology probably started in 1935 when Stein and Leventhal first described the surgical treatment of a group of women with polycystic ovaries by wedge resection. This is quite a major operation, involving the opening of the abdomen and the surgical removal of a wedge from each ovary. Stein and Leventhal reported that, following surgery, most of these women went on to menstruate regularly and that most of those who wanted to conceive did so.

Wedge resection continued to be used until clomiphene citrate became available in 1961 and the gonadotrophins in 1963. Until then, it was the only treatment for women with polycystic ovary syndrome who were anovulatory. Its disadvantage, apart from the fact that it is a major surgical procedure, was that it often led to adhesions around the tubes and ovaries. These adhesions sometimes resulted in the ovulatory infertility being treated successfully but becoming superseded by tubal infertility. With the introduction of the new medical treatments, wedge resection of the ovary became obsolete and rarely used.

During the 1980s, the use of keyhole surgery (laparoscopy) became popular. This enabled a telescope to be inserted through the navel to allow direct visualization of the pelvic and abdominal cavities and for surgical procedures to be carried out through small incisions. Laparoscopy has now become a routine procedure, not only for gynaecological treatment, but also for operations such as the removal of the gall bladder.

The technique of laparoscopy

The technique of endoscopy was developed as a minimally invasive procedure to allow the inspection of the internal organs with telescopic instruments. It originated in Germany in 1901 with a report of the endoscopic inspection of the abdomen of a dog. Although subsequently there were isolated reports of the use of this technique, it was revolutionized when it became possible to transmit 'cool' light from a distant source down fine glass fibres (fibreoptics). There was very little interest in laparoscopy in the UK until the 1960s when Dr Steptoe (of in-vitro fertilization fame) started to publicize its possible use in gynaecology.

Laparoscopy has been used routinely in gynaecology for the last 30 years. It enables the gynaecological organs to be inspected, procedures such as sterilization and removal of ectopic pregnancies to be carried out, and conditions such as pelvic adhesions and endometriosis to be treated. Its use is also widespread in general surgery, with the laparoscopic removal of the gall bladder being one of the great advances of the 1990s.

The technique requires admission to a hospital or day-surgery centre where general anaesthesia is administered. The first step is to introduce a special, guarded, fine needle (known as a Verres needle) under the belly button. The needle is designed so that its sharp end protrudes whilst there is resistance, but as soon as it passes through firm tissue, a rounded, guarded end protrudes. This minimizes the risk of damaging any of the organs within the abdomen. Carbon dioxide gas is then infused through the needle to distend the abdominal wall. The pressure

84

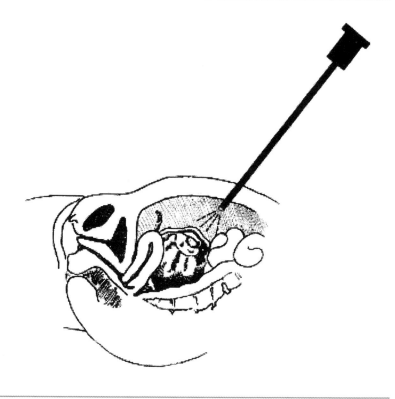

Figure 11.1 The principle of laparoscopy.

of the gas within the system is measured, so that it will become apparent if the needle is not in the right position. Once the abdominal cavity is safely distended, another sharp tubular instrument (between 5 and 10 mm in diameter) is introduced into the cavity of the abdomen (the intraperitoneal space). The sharp, inner part of the instrument is then removed and replaced by a telescope and, when a light source is attached, the pelvic organs can be inspected. To make it even easier to see, a small television camera is attached to the telescope, and pictures are relayed to a television monitor in the operating theatre. Other specialized instruments can also be inserted, such as laparoscopic scissors, forceps and insulated needles that conduct electricity to seal the ends of bleeding blood vessels etc. (Figure 11.1).

GENERAL COMPLICATIONS OF LAPAROSCOPY

There are complications of laparoscopy, but fortunately these are rare. As with any operation performed using an anaesthetic, a skilled, experienced anaesthetist is present in the operating theatre throughout surgery to monitor the patient.

Although a rare complication, it is possible for the Verres needle to cause damage to the internal organs as it is introduced. This risk is reduced with the use of a special retractable, blunt needle. There is also the possibility of the needle being introduced into a blood vessel, but, again, this is a very rare complication. If it does occur, the carbon dioxide gas used to distend the abdomen may enter the circulation and result in gas embolism, which is a potentially fatal condition. Rapid diagnosis of this complication by the anaesthetist and immediate resuscitation are essential.

It is also possible for the abdominal organs or a blood vessel to be damaged as the telescope or auxiliary instruments are introduced and, in order to minimize this risk, other instruments are introduced under direct visualization once the telescope has been inserted.

Other complications may occur during intra-abdominal laparoscopic surgery. For example, if scissors are used, there is the risk of cutting adjoining tissues; when an electric current or laser energy is used, there is a risk of thermal damage to the adjoining tissues. (Diathermy or electrocautery involves the passage of an electric current down a pair of insulated forceps. Laser treatment also involves the use of heat energy to burn away some of the surface cysts.) Of course, great care is taken to avoid these complications, but even so, problems can still occasionally occur. The risk of complications is less than 1%, and therefore 99% of women have uneventful procedures.

Laparoscopic ovarian cautery

During the 1970s and 1980s, various workers (mainly in France) reported that biopsy of the ovaries of women with polycystic ovary syndrome sometimes led to them becoming ovulatory.

It was not until the 1980s that a Scandinavian, Dr Gjonnaes, reported his experience of using laparoscopic burning by electrical cautery of polycystic ovaries (to drain and destroy 10-20 of the surface cysts), which resulted in ovulation rates of 92% and pregnancy rates of nearly 70%. By 1989, Dr Gjonnaes had reported on almost 100 women he had treated in this way. This resulted in a fresh look at the surgical treatment of polycystic ovary syndrome. Numerous publications appeared during the 1990s that showed ovulation rates of over 70% and pregnancy rates of about 50% following laparoscopic surgery.

There is still concern about causing adhesions, but these seem to be less common and certainly less severe than those resulting from wedge resection, and do not affect subsequent pregnancy rates. It has also been noted in some of the studies that the risk of miscarriage of pregnancies achieved after ovarian cautery is reduced from the raised rate of women with polycystic ovaries to that of the normal population.

Sometimes, rather than cauterizing the ovaries with an electric current, laser therapy is used. (However, laser treatment is more complicated and requires expensive and complex equipment and special training, whereas electrocautery can be performed by any competent gynaecologist.) There is no suggestion that the ovulatory rates are higher or the adhesion rates lower with laser treatment compared to simple electrocautery.

COMPLICATIONS

The complications of ovarian cautery include the risks associated with the general anaesthesia. There is also the theoretical concern that, should the thermal damage be too extensive, ovarian atrophy leading to premature menopause may result. However, there is no documented evidence of ovarian atrophy occurring as a result of this treatment.

Conclusions

Although surgical treatment to induce ovulation does have a place, it is a second-line treatment for use only if oral treatment (with clomiphene citrate alone followed by clomiphene and metformin) has been unsuccessful.

How surgical treatment works is not understood. However, as the causes of polycystic ovaries are not understood, this is no surprise. The advantages of a laparoscopic surgical method are that it eliminates the risk of hyperstimulation and multiple pregnancies; multiple ovulations will result from a single cycle of treatment; the pregnancy rate is good; and there is a lower spontaneous abortion rate. Furthermore, the intensity of monitoring and high cost of treatment with gonadotrophins are avoided.

As many women who fail to conceive on clomiphene citrate need to have a diagnostic laparoscopy to assess their pelvis prior to gonadotrophin ovulation induction, it seems reasonable to combine this surgical procedure with ovarian cautery. If ovarian cautery is not followed by ovulation and pregnancy, it is still possible to move on to gonadotrophin ovulation induction. A recent review of all the papers that have looked at comparisons of injections and laparoscopic ovarian cautery showed that the outcomes for the two treatments were comparable.

As far as the other problems of polycystic ovary syndrome such as insulin resistance and increased secretion of androgens are concerned, there is no evidence to suggest that these are reversed by ovarian cautery.

A recent study in Australia comparing the cost of typical cycles of gonadotrophin ovulation induction to that of ovarian electrocautery found that, for insured patients, the cost of laparoscopic cautery was slightly less than that of one cycle of ovulation induction. Therefore, as the cautery usually results in several ovulations, it is more cost-effective as a second choice of treatment if treatment with clomiphene citrate is unsuccessful.

Twelve

In-vitro fertilization

It needs to be emphasized from the outset that most women who have polycystic ovary syndrome will not need in-vitro fertilization (IVF) treatment. The basic reproductive problem with polycystic ovary syndrome is the lack of ovulation and, in more than 90% of patients, this can be overcome by ovulation induction with tablets, injections or ovarian cautery. For the small proportion of women for whom a pregnancy does not result, there are either factors accounting for their subfertility, or that of their partner, or they suffer from unexplained subfertility. Those women who appear normal but fail to conceive despite six ovulations may be recommended to enter an IVF programme.

UNEXPLAINED SUBFERTILITY

Unexplained subfertility is a condition in which the requirements for a pregnancy are present - that is, the woman ovulates, her fallopian tubes are patent and her pelvis is reasonably normal, and she has a male partner with adequate sperm - but she still does not conceive. In the general population, there are many couples who suffer from unexplained subfertility and who may wish to consider IVF.

In-vitro fertilization for infertility in women

IVF was initially developed in the 1970s to overcome tubal disease. The principle of treatment is that hormones (similar to those used for ovulation induction) are administered in higher doses. In contrast to ovulation induction, in which the aim is to produce two or three follicles, the aim of IVF is to produce many more, probably 10-20.

There are various regimens used to induce controlled ovarian hyperstimulation, and most of these now involve the use of a gonadotrophin-releasing hormone (GnRH) agonist. This hormone is similar to the GnRH that stimulates follicle-stimulating hormone (FSH) and luteinizing hormone (LH) in the normal cycle (see page 9), but the analogue is responsible for inhibiting the release of FSH and LH during the IVF cycle. The advantage of its use is that it prevents spontaneous ovulation before the eggs are collected. It can be administered either as a nasal spray or as an injection. When the ovarian follicles have matured, as assessed by rising levels of oestrogen hormone in the blood and ultrasound confirmation of their growth, human chorionic gonadotrophin (HCG) is administered. Then, rather than the couple having intercourse at home, a surgical procedure is performed to retrieve the eggs 36 hours later. This is usually done in an operating theatre or a procedure room and some form of intravenous sedation is used to eliminate any pain involved. The procedure is performed through the vagina; the follicles visible to ultrasound are aspirated and the fluid is removed and sent to the laboratory.

About 70% of ovulatory-sized follicles will yield mature oocytes. Sperm is then provided by the male partner or, occasionally, if he is sterile, donor sperm is used. The eggs are either mixed together with the sperm if the sperm quality is normal or a single sperm is injected into each egg if the sperm quality is poor. This latter technique is known as micro-injection or intracytoplasmic sperm injection (ICSI). The egg and the sperm are then allowed to grow in an incubator, which is a type of 'oven' in which the temperature, gas concentrations and humidity are controlled. They grow in a solution of culture medium, which mimics the natural environment within the body. Usually, 60-70% of mature oocytes fertilize and form early embryos. The embryos are allowed to grow in culture for a day or two before being transferred into the uterine cavity of the woman.

In the early days, IVF was quite time consuming, but most protocols are now streamlined, with minimal time having to be taken off work, and the woman only has to attend the IVF clinic on a few occasions.

EMBRYO TRANSFER PROCEDURE
The embryo transfer procedure is relatively simple and resembles a smear test (with about the same degree of discomfort). A speculum is inserted through the vagina so that the neck of the womb (the cervix) can be seen clearly. A fine tube is then passed through the opening of the uterus into the uterine cavity, and the embryos (usually two or three) are injected in a small volume of culture medium.

Pregnancy rates vary, depending on numerous factors such as the woman's age, the reason for the subfertility and the condition of her pelvis, but rates in the region of 25% per cycle are average.

The IVF process is summarized in Figure 12.1 (see page 92).

EMBRYO FREEZING
Any embryos that are not transferred are allowed to grow for another day or so. Those that look strong enough to survive freezing and thawing are then frozen and stored in liquid nitrogen. These stored embryos allow further IVF treatments to take place without the additional cost and discomfort of stimulation, egg collection and fertilization. About two-thirds of frozen embryos survive and can be transferred. As long as about half the cells of an embryo survive the freezing and thawing process, the embryo is considered to be potentially alive and well, and can be transferred.

As women with polycystic ovaries usually produce large numbers of eggs, the use of embryo freezing is very relevant. Because of the potential risks of ovarian hyperstimulation syndrome (see page 96) in women with polycystic ovaries, it is of benefit to be able to have several attempts at transfer (using frozen-thawed embryos) with minimal attempts at stimulation.

1. hyperstimulation

2. monitoring

3. oocyte collection

4. *in vitro* fertilisation

5. embryo culture

6. embryo transfer

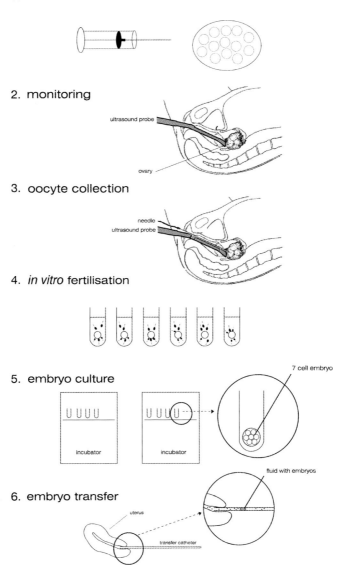

Figure 12.1 The IVF process.

THE PROCESS OF FROZEN EMBRYO TRANSFER IN WOMEN WITH POLYCYSTIC OVARY SYNDROME

Normally, the transfer of frozen embryos is a very simple procedure. All that is required is to monitor the woman's cycle and replace embryos on the appropriate day after ovulation. In straightforward cycles, no other hormone treatment is necessary. The problem for women who have polycystic ovary syndrome is that they often do not ovulate regularly, thus making the determination of the time of ovulation more difficult. Furthermore, even if the trigger for ovulation (the rise in HCG) is detected, there is no guarantee that adequate ovulation will occur. Consequently, appropriate hormone secretion with normal development of the uterine lining may not take place.

The transferred frozen-thawed embryos depend on adequate development of the uterine lining following ovulation, and inadequate ovulation may result in an underdeveloped uterine lining and a decreased chance of successful implantation. To avoid this problem, hormone treatment is often used for frozen embryo transfer cycles in women with polycystic ovary syndrome. Either clomiphene can be used to regulate ovulation, or artificial hormone replacement treatment can be given with oestrogen tablets and progesterone pessaries or injections to stimulate the laying down of the uterine lining and to make it receptive for the transferred embryos.

In-vitro fertilization for subfertility in men

Although IVF was developed for the treatment of tubal infertility, it was realized in the mid-1980s that it is a very good way of overcoming male subfertility as well. Today, the main reason for undergoing IVF treatment for one in three couples is male subfertility, and up to 20% of the female partners of these men have polycystic ovaries.

Moderate male subfertility can be treated with standard IVF, but, if there are significant sperm abnormalities, the micro-injection technique (in which a single sperm is injected into an oocyte) needs to be carried out. This has now been practised for a decade and has resulted in a tremendous improvement in prognosis for subfertile males. In some situations, even men who do not produce any sperm by ejaculation can undergo a surgical procedure in which sperm are removed from the testicle and subsequently used for IVF. This means that sperm can often be removed from the testicle of a man who does not produce any sperm by ejaculation (because of an outflow blockage) or who has a very low rate of production.

Response of the polycystic ovary to stimulation for in-vitro fertilization

Women with polycystic ovary syndrome respond to stimulation differently from women with normal ovaries. There are two possible responses.

1. Often, the women seem to respond very vigorously, with a significant risk of ovarian hyperstimulation and cyst formation.
2. Alternatively, some women with polycystic ovary syndrome will be resistant and do not respond to routine doses of FSH.

An excessive response is probably due to the presence of many partially developed follicles in polycystic ovaries that are ready to stimulate and give rise to a multifollicular response with rapidly escalating levels of oestrogens. There are several causes of an excessive response.

1. As mentioned above, there are many follicles present, which may all respond once FSH is administered. Under the influence of LH, the cells in the ovary convert the male hormones androstenedione and testosterone - the circulating levels of which are raised in women with polycystic ovary syndrome - into oestradiol, thus rapidly raising the level of oestrogen. This rapid rise in the level of oestradiol further sensitizes the follicle to FSH.
2. Insulin acts as a co-gonadotrophin, i.e. it enhances the effect of the gonadotrophins, and women with polycystic ovary syndrome may have higher levels of insulin than normal.

3. During normal ovulation, blood is diverted to the ovary that is ovulating and, within that ovary, to the leading follicle. Women with polycystic ovaries have increased levels of vascular epithelial growth factor (VEGF), both before and during hormonal stimulation. This widespread distribution of VEGF enables blood to flow past all the small follicles, which consequently develop quickly and produce large amounts of oestrogen.

Counselling couples about the risks of in-vitro fertilization

The first part of counselling is pre-pregnancy counselling. It is always advisable for an obese woman with polycystic ovary syndrome to lose weight *before* embarking on a pregnancy. This is beneficial in decreasing the risk of developing raised blood pressure during the confinement. Once pregnancy is achieved, maintaining or even losing weight will not decrease the risk of high blood pressure.

Women with polycystic ovary syndrome also have an increased miscarriage rate. This is probably due to their raised levels of basal LH, which seem to have deleterious effects on both the oocyte and the endometrium. There is some debate about whether using GnRH agonists, which decrease the levels of LH in the blood prior to IVF, has a significant effect on this.

Women with polycystic ovaries also seem to have an increased risk of hyperstimulation (as discussed above), for which they need to be counselled. They are also at risk of multiple pregnancies, although this risk is no different from that associated with other methods of assisted reproductive technology. However, one reassuring fact is that the incidence of congenital malformations in children born to women with polycystic ovaries is no greater than that for the 'normal' population.

Ovarian hyperstimulation syndrome

Ovarian hyperstimulation syndrome (OHSS) is briefly discussed in Chapter 10 as it can arise as a complication of ovulation induction. However, it is the most serious - and possibly life-threatening - potential complication of IVF and therefore is dealt with in more detail here. OHSS is particularly relevant for women with polycystic ovaries, as they are far more likely to experience this complication. The most important aspect of its management is to try to avoid it. Women who are known to have polycystic ovaries are given a smaller dose of FSH than other women. Also, monitoring of oestrogen levels during stimulation allows the administration of FSH to be limited in an attempt to limit ovarian stimulation. If, despite these measures, there is a serious risk of ovarian hyperstimulation, the cycle may be abandoned and no HCG administered, as it is believed that HCG is the trigger for OHSS. It is usual practice to continue the administration of the GnRH antagonist (using a nasal spray or injections) for a few extra days. However, if the hyperstimulation is not significant enough to cancel the cycle, it may be decided to collect the eggs, but not to contemplate embryo transfer. This is because, if pregnancy does occur, the ßHCG secreted by the early embryo aggravates the severity of OHSS. In this case, all the embryos can be frozen and replaced as thawed embryos, two or three at a time, in subsequent cycles.

A new experimental treatment that is being evaluated in some IVF units is the collection of 'immature eggs' from women with a risk of hyperstimulation without administering the HCG to induce maturation. It is believed that, if HCG is not administered, the risk of OHSS is minimalized. However, this treatment is still experimental, and the maturation of immature eggs in the laboratory still has a fairly low success rate.

The first signs of OHSS are bloating, abdominal pain and nausea. Abdominal ultrasound shows enlarged ovaries, with free fluid in the pelvic cavity and abdomen (called ascites) and sometimes fluid collection around the lungs (pleural effusion). Sometimes, difficulty with breathing and shortness of breath are experienced. There are metabolic changes, with fluid escaping from the circulation into the body cavities, resulting in thickening of the blood and an increased risk of blood clotting.

Many patients only develop mild symptoms of distension and discomfort, which can be controlled by pain relief at home. Successful monitoring can be carried out with daily weighing to see if fluid is being retained and measurement of the woman's abdominal girth. If nausea, pain relief or shortness of breath requires hospitalization, intravenous fluids are usually administered. The blood-thinning medication heparin is often used to decrease the risk of clotting and, occasionally, if the abdomen is very distended and uncomfortable, some of the excess fluid is withdrawn with a needle under local anaesthesia. Although this relieves the symptoms, the fluid often rapidly re-accumulates.

OHSS is usually self-limiting, and resolves by the next menstrual period. Often, however, it is associated with a conception, especially if there is a multiple pregnancy. When this occurs, the symptoms may persist (although in a less severe form) for some weeks.

Thirteen

Risk factors for pregnant women with polycystic ovary syndrome

Introduction

It has long been recognized that women with a history of treatment for subfertility have higher pregnancy complications than normal. Miscarriages seem to occur more often, as do pregnancies in the fallopian tube (ectopic pregnancies). Bleeding from the placenta and high blood pressure are more common, as are prematurity, lower birth weight and, as a result, perinatal mortality and morbidity.

These problems can, in part, be attributed to the facts that these women are often older than other women becoming pregnant and are having their first pregnancy. Also, multiple pregnancies are more common after treatments that require superovulation. The incidence of early pregnancy loss seems to be 15% amongst women with polycystic ovary syndrome and about 1% have recurrent episodes of miscarriage. Women with polycystic ovary syndrome seem to be represented more frequently than normal amongst patients experiencing recurrent pregnancy loss, and it is thought that this is associated with higher basal luteinizing hormone (LH) levels. The mechanism of action may be associated with the quality of the oocytes produced, or even with the endometrial lining.

Miscarriage

It has been noted by some doctors that women with polycystic ovary syndrome who are lean have an increased probability of miscarriage, but other studies have reported higher miscarriage rates among obese women with polycystic ovaries. Exercise and lifestyle modification programmes (see Chapter 7) have reportedly been associated with decreased miscarriage rates. Also, it is not clear whether the altered insulin sensitivity associated with a raised level of insulin may play a role in the pregnancy loss associated with polycystic ovary syndrome.

Whatever the reasons, there is widespread agreement that there is an association between polycystic ovary syndrome and early pregnancy loss and that this is most marked in women who have high levels of LH. However, the picture is somewhat complicated by the varying aspects of polycystic ovary syndrome and also by the different diagnostic criteria employed in various studies. It would appear that the presence of a raised early follicular LH level, an ultrasound diagnosis of polycystic ovary syndrome, obesity, insulin resistance and increased male hormone levels may also, singly or in combination, be associated with an increased miscarriage risk.

As already mentioned, ovarian hyperstimulation syndrome (OHSS - see page 96) is more common if a pregnancy results. This is thought to be due to the rising human chorionic gonadotrophin (HCG) level stimulating the remaining corpora lutea to secrete high levels of oestrogen. Although this exacerbates the OHSS, there is no long-term ill-effect on the pregnancy. There is a higher incidence of OHSS in multiple pregnancies and it is only as a result of the multiple pregnancy that the risks are increased.

Although early reports of ovulation induction suggested that tubal ectopic pregnancies were more common, large, long-term studies have shown that there is no increased risk, either in polycystic ovary syndrome alone or after treatment with ovulation induction drugs.

Gestational diabetes

Gestational diabetes (diabetes of pregnancy) occurs often enough during the pregnancies of women with polycystic ovary syndrome for routine screening to be recommended at 28 weeks of gestation. If gestational diabetes continues undetected, the baby grows extremely quickly and becomes very large, the perinatal outcome is poor and the delivery is difficult. In the worst-case scenario, unexplained stillbirth can occur.

At least in some studies, the incidence of gestational diabetes amongst infertile women with polycystic ovary syndrome who conceive either spontaneously or following ovulation induction treatment has been reported to be no higher than that of the general population.

Although obesity itself is a risk factor for gestational diabetes, there seems to be no difference in the incidence of gestational diabetes of obese and lean polycystic ovary syndrome patients.

It is essential that any woman with polycystic ovary syndrome who conceives should undergo appropriate tests for glucose levels. If she is found to have gestational diabetes, her blood sugar must be controlled by diet and, sometimes, insulin. Even with better control of blood sugar levels during the pregnancy, complications are more common.

Pregnancy-induced hypertension

This is defined as hypertension (high blood pressure) that develops as a consequence of pregnancy and regresses after delivery. If associated with the presence of protein in the urine, it is usually called pre-eclampsia. Pre-eclampsia can be mild or severe. The fetal effects of pregnancy-induced hypertension include intra-uterine growth restriction (small, skinny babies), a higher rate of bleeding from the placenta (abruptio-placenta) and prematurity secondary to early intervention for maternal complications. Pre-eclampsia is still a major cause of maternal morbidity and mortality.

Several studies have reported that women with polycystic ovary syndrome have a higher incidence of pregnancy-induced hypertension, which appears to be independent of both obesity and gestational diabetes. It is thought that insulin resistance and high levels of insulin may have a role in the development of these complications. Again, the blood pressure levels of women with polycystic ovary syndrome who conceive after treatment, or even spontaneously, should be screened and monitored regularly.

Conclusions

Fortunately, most women with polycystic ovary syndrome conceive either spontaneously or after appropriate treatment. Of those who become pregnant, most will have an uncomplicated pregnancy and a live birth. However, women with all forms of polycystic ovary syndrome have an increased risk of pregnancy loss compared to the general population and an increased chance of a multiple pregnancy should conception follow ovulation induction treatment. They also have an increased risk of gestational diabetes and pregnancy-induced hypertension. These risks all result in a poorer outcome of pregnancy for these women, some of which may be decreased by losing weight prior to becoming pregnant. However, the long-term benefits of treatments with respect to later pregnancy complications remain unknown.

F o u r t e e n

Contraception

Introduction

Whereas many women with polycystic ovary syndrome consult a gynaecologist because of their inability to conceive and because they have irregular periods, there are many women with polycystic ovaries who do not wish to become pregnant and who require contraception. Despite the fact that irregular menstruation makes it less likely that a woman will conceive, women with irregular cycles are still potentially fertile and need to use contraception. Even women who are experiencing a total lack of periods may ovulate occasionally, without any warning or symptoms. If unprotected intercourse occurs at the time when an oocyte is being released, pregnancy can occur. It is reasonable to assume that a woman who only ovulates infrequently is less at risk of becoming pregnant than someone who ovulates regularly, but she is still at risk. It is not unusual for a gynaecologist to see women who have not had a period for some months but who are pregnant. As menstruation only occurs 2 weeks after ovulation if conception does not occur, there may be no warning that ovulation has taken place. If the woman does not experience the signs of early pregnancy such as morning sickness, the pregnancy may continue unrecognized for weeks or months.

Therefore, the message is that even one ovulation may result in pregnancy, and if a woman does not want to become pregnant but is planning to be sexually active, she needs contraception.

102

The choice of the method a particular woman uses will depend on a number of factors, and all the methods available are potential options for women with polycystic ovaries or polycystic ovary syndrome.

Oral contraceptives

The contraceptive of choice for most women with polycystic ovary syndrome is a combined oral contraceptive ('the pill'). These pills consist of an oestrogen and a progestogen. Progestogens are synthetic hormones with a progesterone-like action that have been developed because progesterone itself is not active when taken by mouth. Almost all the progestogens in the various pill preparations are derivatives of the male hormone testosterone. This is not good news for women with polycystic ovaries, as they already have excessive amounts of circulating male-type hormones. The only currently available oral contraceptive that does not contain a testosterone derivative is the one that contains cyproterone acetate (see Chapter 9) as the progestogen. This is called Diane® (Schering) and contains 2 mg of cyproterone acetate with 35 µg of the oestrogen oestradiol. It is the first choice for women with polycystic ovaries. In Australia, this pill is not on the Pharmaceutical Benefits Scheme and is more expensive than others.

Another approach for women with polycystic ovaries is to use an 'oestrogen-dominant pill', i.e. a pill with a higher oestrogen:progestogen ratio. Oestrogen-dominant pills are 'biphasic': for the first half of the cycle, a pill with a relatively low level of progestogen (levonorgestrel) is taken; for the second half of the cycle, this is replaced by a pill with a higher level of progestogen. A pill containing 50 µg of oestrogen is also taken throughout the entire cycle.

The third option is to use a 'third-generation' progestogen pill, which, as its name suggests, is the most recently developed of this type of contraceptive. The third-generation pills have less male hormone activity than the 'second-generation' progestogens and are therefore less harmful.

The oestrogenic pills also have a beneficial effect on the skin and, to a small degree, on hair growth.

The only theoretical reasons for women with polycystic ovaries to avoid the use of oral contraceptives are that these pills also induce insulin resistance to a small degree and affect cholesterol in an unfavourable way. However, these disadvantages may be outweighed by the benefits - especially the benefits of regulating the menstrual periods, preventing the action of unopposed oestrogens on the endometrium (which increase the risk of endometrial cancer in women with polycystic ovaries, see page 39) and providing the most effective form of reversible contraception. Oral contraceptives should therefore be considered by young women with polycystic ovaries.

The only other concern about the use of oral contraceptives by young women before they have children is that taking them for a prolonged period before the first pregnancy has been reported as a risk factor for breast cancer, although the risk is only slightly raised.

THE MINIPILL
The disadvantages of the minipill are that it does not control the menstrual cycle (bleeding remaining frequent and irregular, or absent) and it has to be taken at about the same time each day. Also, although there is no reason why a woman with polycystic ovaries could not use the minipill, it does not have as great a benefit as the combined pill. However, although the progestogen in the minipill is of the androgen type, it is not present in sufficient quantities to aggravate symptoms.

Progestogen implants

The new progestogen implant Implanon® (Organon) can be used by women with polycystic ovaries, but it is less reliable at regulating the menstrual cycles than the pill. It does have an effect on the uterine lining, and no deleterious effects on other biochemical profiles. These implants are effective for up to 3 years, and present another useful contraceptive option.

Intrauterine devices

Intrauterine devices are not a good option for women who have not already had a child, but they are useful for family spacing or for those who do not wish to have any more children. Either copper-containing or progestogen-releasing devices are suitable, as the progestogen is not absorbed into the system, but acts locally on the uterine lining alone.

With respect to polycystic ovary syndrome, copper-containing devices are neutral, having no beneficial or deleterious effects. They are highly effective (second only to hormonal methods), and their only associated increased risk is that of pelvic inflammatory disease for the first month after insertion. Women using intrauterine devices should be in a mutually monogamous relationship in order to minimize the risk of pelvic inflammatory disease.

The progestogen-releasing intrauterine system Mirena® (Schering) has a beneficial effect on the uterine lining and should also decrease the incidence of heavy periods.

Barrier methods

These include condoms, diaphragms, cervical caps, female condoms and spermicides. Although they are all less effective than hormonal methods, the fact that women with polycystic ovary syndrome may be less fertile may balance the risk to some degree. The use of condoms is also beneficial in decreasing the risk of sexually transmitted infections. None of these methods has any effect on the symptoms or complications of polycystic ovaries.

Natural methods

The principle behind natural methods of contraception is that intercourse is avoided during a woman's 'fertile phase'. The problem that women with polycystic ovary syndrome are faced with is that, if their ovulation and menstrual cycles are irregular and unpredictable, it is far more difficult to determine when their 'fertile phase' occurs. Using the 'rhythm method' (which depends on predicting the possible days of ovulation on the basis of the length of previous cycles) is virtually impossible for women with irregular cycles. Even the Billings mucus method (which depends on detecting the 'fertile mucus' as a sign of imminent ovulation) is far more difficult for women with irregular cycles.

Sterilization

For those women with polycystic ovaries who do not wish to have any more children, sterilization can be carried out. Polycystic ovary syndrome has no effect on sterilization, nor does the sterilization procedure affect polycystic ovaries.

A p p e n d i x I

Body mass index (BMI) table

Height (feet and inches)	5.0	5.1	5.2	5.3	5.4	5.5	5.6	5.7	5.8	5.9	5.10	5.11
Height (cm)	152	155	157	160	163	165	167	170	173	175	177	180
50 kg	**21.8**	20.8	20.1	19.7	18.9	18.4	17.8	17.3	16.8	16.3	16.0	15.5
55 kg	**23.8**	**22.9**	**22.1**	**21.4**	20.9	20.2	19.7	19.1	18.3	18.0	17.7	17.0
60 kg	**25.8**	**25.0**	**24.2**	**23.5**	**22.8**	**22.1**	**21.4**	20.8	20.1	19.7	19.2	18.6
65 kg	28.1	26.9	26.1	**25.3**	**24.8**	**23.9**	**23.3**	**22.6**	**21.8**	**21.2**	20.8	20.0
70 kg	30.3	29.1	28.2	27.3	26.7	**25.8**	**25.0**	**24.2**	**23.4**	**22.9**	**22.3**	**21.8**
75 kg	32.5	31.1	30.1	29.2	28.5	27.4	26.8	26.0	**25.2**	**24.6**	**24.0**	**23.1**
80 kg	34.7	33.1	32.3	31.2	30.4	29.3	28.6	27.7	26.8	26.2	**25.2**	**24.8**
85 kg	36.8	35.1	34.4	33.1	32.4	31.2	30.1	29.5	28.6	27.8	27.1	**25.2**
90 kg	39.0	37.3	36.1	35.0	34.3	33.0	32.2	31.2	30.2	29.4	28.6	27.8
95 kg	41.0	39.5	38.2	37.0	36.0	35.0	34.1	33.0	31.9	31.1	30.3	29.3
100 kg	43.2	41.5	40.1	39.0	38.0	37.0	35.8	34.6	33.5	32.8	31.8	31.0

The figures in the table apply to both men and women.
Normal levels are given in bold print.

Appendix II

Instructions for the collection of a specimen of semen

1. Before producing a semen sample for analysis, it is requested that you abstain from sexual intercourse for 2-3 days. The number of days of sexual abstinence will be recorded on the day of your appointment to allow an assessment to be made of the quality of your sperm.

2. The specimen should be collected by masturbation into a sterile container labelled with your name and the date. If you have any problems producing the sample by masturbation, it can be collected during intercourse by using a special semen collection device, which is available from most semen laboratories.

3. After the specimen has been produced at home, it must be delivered to the andrology laboratory as soon as possible. The sample should be kept warm, at body temperature, during transport, e.g. in a coat pocket. Some laboratories provide a facility on site to produce a semen sample and, if relevant, you should enquire about this when you make your appointment.

4. Sterile specimen containers should be collected from the laboratory or your doctor or may be purchased from a local chemist.

5. Please be careful not to use any commercial lubricants as these may affect the quality of your sperm. If in doubt, check with the andrology laboratory.

6. It is very important to collect the total ejaculate, as the majority of sperm may be present in the first part of it. If some of the semen sample has been lost, inform the laboratory when you deliver it.

7. On the day of your appointment, please inform the laboratory staff if you are taking any medication. It is also important to inform them if you have had any recent fevers, infections or any other illness, as these may affect your sperm quality.

8. At least two semen samples are often required for analysis because the quality may vary.

When your semen specimen is delivered to the laboratory, the volume of the ejaculate will be measured. Three further parameters are then studied in detail:

1. the sperm concentration (i.e. the number of sperm present in the sample),
2. the mobility of the spermatazoa (medically, this is called their motility): both the percentage of sperm moving and their quality (i.e. their 'friskiness'),
3. the percentage of sperm with a normal shape.

There are various ways of measuring the mobility of sperm, including assessing their motile index or measuring the percentage of sperm that are moving forwards. The shape of sperm varies, and, like people, sperm come in all shapes and sizes. Those that have a completely normal head, body and tail are considered 'normal', whereas the others are considered 'abnormal'. How sperm shape is assessed varies from laboratory to laboratory.

Usually, the results of the semen analysis will be sent to your doctor, who will discuss them with you at your next consultation.

Appendix III
Instructions for keeping a temperature chart to detect ovulation

The progesterone released after ovulation has the effect of raising the body temperature, which can therefore be used as a 'marker' for ovulation. Although this rise in temperature is quite small, it can be detected as a slight increase in the basal temperature on waking in the morning.

All that is needed to compile a basal body temperature chart is the chart itself (see opposite) and a thermometer. A mercury thermometer should be shaken each night before going to bed. A digital thermometer just needs to be placed on the bedside table.

The days of the menstrual cycle should also be recorded, using a cross for the days of menstruation and a tick for the days of 'spotting'. By convention, the morning of the first day on which a period occurs is recorded as day 1 of the cycle. The date (day and month) should also be noted on the chart. Each morning on waking up, the thermometer should be placed under the tongue - a digital thermometer until it bleeps or a mercury thermometer for 3 minutes. It is important that the temperature is taken *immediately* on awakening.

The temperature must be recorded accurately and indicated on the chart by a dot. At the end of the month, the dots can be joined together to show a clear pattern on the chart.

Days on which intercourse takes place should also be recorded on the chart, and a new chart should be started when the next menstrual cycle begins.

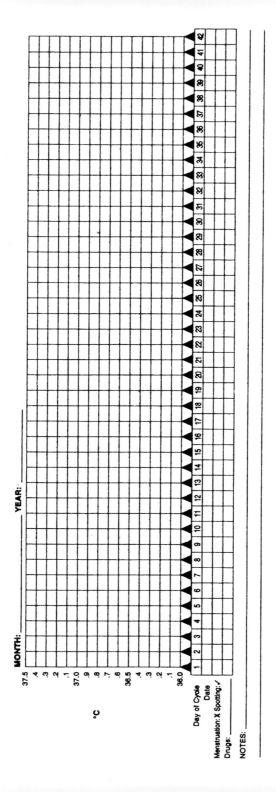

111

A p p e n d i x I V

Ovulation induction:
questions and answers*

1. What are the medicines used for ovulation induction?

Before commencing treatment, you need to have a series of hormone injections of two types: follicle-stimulating hormone (FSH) and luteinizing hormone (LH). These usually come in a powder form, and the boxes contain both the active powder and water in which to dissolve the powder immediately prior to injection.

FSH is now made in a recombinant form, i.e. it is a synthetic, chemically engineered medicine that mimics the action of naturally produced FSH. It is approved by the Australian Health Department and has been in use since 1996. The dose of FSH is measured in international units (IU/mL). It is either Gonal F® (Serono), which comes in 75-IU or 150-IU ampoules, or Puregon® (Organon), which comes in 50-IU, 100-IU or 200-IU ampoules. It is now also available in solution.

The second type of hormone is human chorionic gonadotrophin (HCG), identical in action to LH, which is derived and purified from the urine of pregnant women. It is available either as Pregnyl® (Organon), which comes in 1500-IU ampoules or Profasi® (Serono), which is in 5000-IU ampoules.

In Australia, the hormones are issued by the Health Department on an authority prescription, which needs to be written by your specialist and then sent to the Health Department for approval. After approval, the prescription is sent to you and you need to have it filled by your chemist. When dispensed, the powder form of the hormones needs to be kept in the body of a domestic refrigerator.

---

*   Modified from Monash Ovulation Induction Service, Questions and Answers for Ovulation Induction.

Sometimes, human menopausal gonadotrophin (HMG) is used, which is derived and purified from the urine of post-menopausal women. It has been available since 1963, either as Humegon® (Organon) or Metrodin HP® (Serono). It comes only in powder form.

2. How do I mix and administer the injections?

The injections are available either as a ready-mixed solution or as powder and solvent (solution in which it is to be dissolved).

If in a powder form, both ampoules, the one containing the powder and the one containing the solution, need to be opened by snapping off the top. Draw up the liquid into the syringe, using a 19-gauge (wide-bore) needle, and then transfer this solution into the ampoule containing the powder. The powder will dissolve immediately. Draw the solution back into the syringe and, if more than one ampoule containing powder is needed for the required dose, transfer the made-up solution into the next ampoule, using this to dissolve the second lot of powder. If the preparation is in the solution form, then all you have to do is to suck up the solution into a syringe using the 19-gauge needle.

Attach a 26-gauge (thin) needle, hold the syringe vertically and expel any air. The injection is then ready to give.

To give the injection, choose a site on your abdomen below the belly button. Wipe the injection site with antiseptic, then pinch the skin with one hand pushing the needle in at 90 degrees to its full depth.

Inject all the solution and then quickly remove the needle. Put pressure on the injection site to minimize bleeding and bruising.

Dispose of the used syringe safely.

3. What effect do the injections have?

The main function of follicle-stimulating hormone (FSH) is to stimulate follicle growth in the ovaries. The follicles contain the eggs that are released at ovulation. Daily injections are used to mimic (as closely as possible) the hormones released in the follicular phase (the first half of the normal reproductive cycle). Once the follicles grow to the desired size and the eggs are mature, ovulation is triggered by a single injection of human chorionic gonadotrophin (HCG). Your doctor may also give you smaller doses of HCG for the luteal phase (after ovulation) to support the growth of the endometrium.

4. How is my response to the hormones assessed?

You need to attend the clinic twice weekly (depending on your response) so that the oestrogen level in your blood can be measured, and to have transvaginal ultrasound measurements of your ovarian follicles.

5. Why do I need to have both blood tests and ultrasound procedures performed?

The blood test estimates the amount of specific hormones in the bloodstream. In the first part of the cycle, the blood is tested for oestrogen, the level of which indicates follicle growth. However, this level does not reveal whether one large follicle has developed or many smaller follicles are present. Therefore, an ultrasound is performed to visualize the ovaries so that the number and size of follicles can be estimated.

6. Can my husband/partner come with me to appointments?

Partners are encouraged to attend the clinic. In this way, both members of a couple are informed about the progress of treatment and can support one another.

7. How many cycles of ovulation induction will I need?

The approximate pregnancy rate for the average patient is 20% per cycle. Approximately half the patients who start ovulation induction conceive within three ovulations. Careful reassessment is recommended after three ovulations if a pregnancy has not occurred.

8. Is there anything else we should be doing to maximize our chances of having a child?

It is thought that lifestyle behaviours can have a large impact on the outcome of infertility treatments as well as on general health and well-being.

Lifestyle factors

♦ *Smoking.* Smoking increases the risks of lung, throat, breast and cardiovascular disease. In addition, it has an effect on infertility. It is thought that eggs travel more slowly through the fallopian tube in some women who smoke. The sperm from some male smokers has decreased mobility and therefore the egg and sperm are older (and probably less viable) at the time of fertilization. If you are a smoker, you should ask the clinic nurse or your general practitioner (GP) for a QUIT program.

♦ *Weight management.* Some women who are underweight or overweight can experience difficulty in achieving pregnancy. For some underweight women, the hypothalamus ceases to function, which in turn interrupts the process of ovulation. (The hypothalamus is the part of the brain near the pituitary gland, and is also known as the 'master gland'.)

For some overweight women, excessive production of the hormone *testosterone* causes a hormone imbalance, which in turn interrupts the reproductive cycle. A return to a reasonable weight may assist the process of conception. The clinic nurses can assist you with weight-management advice and support. In addition, a referral to a clinical nutritionist can be arranged.

♦ *Stress relief.* Although stress is not a known cause of infertility, increased stress levels resulting in feelings of being unable to cope do not assist general health and well-being. Methods of relaxation can include recreational sport, exercise and leisure activities. Inappropriate forms of stress relief, such as excessive alcohol intake, drugs etc., may require counselling assistance.

♦ *Alcohol intake.* Excess alcohol is known to have a teratogenic effect on the fetus (i.e. it can cause abnormalities). It is therefore not recommended in pregnancy.

9. Is there any other pregnancy preparation I should attend to?

Research indicates that women who have a diet rich in folic acid are less likely to have babies with neural tube defects, such as spina bifida and anencephaly. All women planning a pregnancy are advised to take folic acid supplementation (0.5 mg per day) prior to becoming pregnant and for the first 3 months of pregnancy. Note: women who take anti-convulsant medication (e.g. Tegretol/Dilantin) should take extra folic acid supplementation under the supervision of their treating physician.

10. I have been told sometimes, when I come to the clinic, that I cannot commence treatment because of a cyst. What is a cyst?

The definition of a cyst is 'a fluid-filled space'. By this definition, therefore, the words follicle and cyst are interchangeable. Every woman normally has tiny cysts in her ovaries. Some women have large cysts present (seen by ultrasound examination) at the beginning of their cycle. When this situation occurs, the woman is advised to wait until the cystic structure has shrunk so that the cysts will not be confused with growing follicles on ultrasound examination.

11. What are the risks and side-effects of ovulation induction?

As far as is known at present, the risks and side-effects of this treatment are as follows.

- *Needle-site discomfort.* Some patients may experience slight irritation or bruising at the site of the injection where the blood test was taken.

- *Abdominal discomfort.* Sometimes, in the last half of a treatment cycle (after ovulation), some women experience a feeling of having a 'bloated' abdomen: this is due to post-ovulation hormone production. When a woman experiences this type of symptom, she is encouraged to take a Panadol tablet and to inform the clinic nurse.

- *Ovarian hyperstimulation syndrome (OHSS).* Hyperstimulation or overstimulation of the ovary may cause the ovaries to swell and become painful. Symptoms of mild hyperstimulation include abdominal bloating, tenderness and nausea. Vomiting and/or diarrhoea may occur when mild to moderate hyperstimulation exists. Severe symptoms of hyperstimulation include breathing difficulties and the presence of fluid in the abdomen, with accompanying medical problems. Careful monitoring during the treatment cycle is undertaken in order to minimize the risk of hyperstimulation occurring.

- *Multiple pregnancy.* Despite the utmost care, there is still an approximately 20% incidence of twins and a 2% incidence of higher-order multiple pregnancies while on this and similar major ovulation induction programmes around the world. Careful monitoring using vaginal ultrasound and blood tests is undertaken to minimize the risk of multiple pregnancy.
- *Cancelled cycle.* Sometimes, during a cycle, the oestrogen level and the ultrasound result indicate that there is a real risk of a high-order multiple pregnancy. In this situation, the health and well-being of the woman may be adversely affected by the risks of ovarian hyperstimulation and/or by the multiple pregnancy itself. Should these signs of a potential risk occur, it will be suggested that the cycle does not continue. The couple will then be advised either to abstain from intercourse or to use a barrier contraceptive. The information concerning the woman's cycle will be used to manage future treatment cycles more effectively.

12. Are there other risks associated with infertility?

There is a slightly increased risk of some gynaecological cancers. Further information about gynaecological cancers can be obtained from your doctor and from the Anti-Cancer Council.

13. I have been told that there is an increased risk of osteoporosis associated with infertility. What can I do to protect myself or at least to minimize the risk?

Some women with medical conditions that result in infertility have an increased risk of osteoporosis. If you do have an increased risk factor, it is advisable to eat a high-calcium diet and to do 2-3 hours of weight-bearing exercise per week, such as walking, running or aerobics.

14. How early can pregnancy be detected?

A blood test is usually performed on the 16th day after the human chorionic gonadotrophin injection is given. The test result often indicates a positive or negative pregnancy result. Sometimes, however, the result is unclear and will be repeated several days later. Even if the pregnancy blood test is positive at 16 days, it is very early and some pregnancies do not become established.

15. What signs and symptoms of pregnancy are usually noticed first?

Many women do not experience any changes in early pregnancy. However, some women experience breast tenderness and slight pain or discomfort in the lower abdomen.

16. What is the procedure when I do become pregnant?

Women with infertility problems have a slightly increased risk of miscarriage and blood tests are therefore done to monitor the progress of the pregnancy. About 4 weeks after ovulation, an ultrasound examination is performed to assess the development of the pregnancy and to determine whether a fetal heart beat is present. At this time, you will be asked where you would like to have your baby, so that the clinic doctor can refer you for obstetric management.

Appendix V
Further reading

Kovacs G, editor. The Polycystic Ovary. Cambridge, UK: Cambridge University Press 2000.
This is the first comprehensive textbook on polycystic ovary syndrome, with each chapter written by the leading world expert.

Wood C, Kovacs G. Infertility, All your Questions Answered. Melbourne, Australia: Hill of Content 1996.

Kovacs G, editor. Polycystic Ovary Syndrome. Cambridge, UK: Cambridge University Press 2000.

Thatcher S. Polycystic Ovary Syndrome. Indianapolis, USA: Perspectives Press 2000.

Cheung T, Harris C. PCOS Diet Book. London, UK: Thorsons Harper Collins. (due for publication August 2002).

Homburg R, editor. Polycystic Ovary Syndrome. London, UK: Martin Dunitz 2001.

Appendix VI

Contact details for
patient support organizations

UK

Verity - The Polycystic Ovaries Self-Help Group
52-54 Featherstone Street
London
EC1Y 8RT
Web site: www.verity-pcos.org.uk
Email: enquiries@verity-pcos.org.uk

USA

PCOS Association
PO Box 80517
Portland, OR 97280
Telephone: (503) 977-6187
Toll Free Information: (877) 775-PCOS
Web site: www.pcosupport.org

Australia

Polycystic Ovarian Syndrome Association of Australia Inc.
PO Box E140
Emerton, NSW 2770
Email: info@posaa.asn.au

Victoria

Polycystic Ovarian Syndrome Association of Victoria
c/o Ms Junelle Rhodes
Telephone: (03) 9776 8352